Reading – Key Ideas and Details
© Mometrix Media - flashcardsecrets.com/teas
ATI TEAS Exam

Describe the process of summarizing.

Visit *mometrix.com/academy* for a related video.
Enter video code: 172903

Reading – Key Ideas and Details
© Mometrix Media - flashcardsecrets.com/teas
ATI TEAS Exam

Describe paraphrasing.

Reading – Key Ideas and Details
© Mometrix Media - flashcardsecrets.com/teas
ATI TEAS Exam

Discuss the process of identifying the logical conclusion given a reading selection.

Reading – Key Ideas and Details
© Mometrix Media - flashcardsecrets.com/teas
ATI TEAS Exam

Describe the process of drawing conclusions.

Reading – Key Ideas and Details
© Mometrix Media - flashcardsecrets.com/teas
ATI TEAS Exam

Describe the process of making inferences from a text.

Visit *mometrix.com/academy* for a related video.
Enter video code: 379203

Reading – Key Ideas and Details
© Mometrix Media - flashcardsecrets.com/teas
ATI TEAS Exam

Describe how context clues help with inference.

Paraphrasing is another method that the reader can use to aid in comprehension. When paraphrasing, one puts what they have read into their words by **rephrasing** what the author has written, or one "translates" all of what the author shared into their words by including as many details as they can.

A helpful tool is the ability to **summarize** the information that you have read in a paragraph or passage format. This process is similar to creating an effective outline. First, a summary should accurately define the **main idea** of the passage though the summary does not need to explain this main idea in exhaustive detail. The summary should continue by laying out the most important **supporting details** or arguments from the passage. All of the significant supporting details should be included, and none of the details included should be irrelevant or insignificant. Also, the summary should accurately report all of these details. Too often, the desire for brevity in a summary leads to the sacrifice of clarity or accuracy. Summaries are often difficult to read because they omit all of the graceful language, digressions, and asides that distinguish great writing. However, an effective summary should contain much the same message as the original text.

A reader should always be drawing conclusions from the text. Sometimes conclusions are implied from written information, and other times the information is **stated directly** within the passage. One should always aim to draw **conclusions** from information stated within a passage, rather than to draw them from mere implications. At times an author may provide some information and then describe a **counterargument**. Readers should be alert for direct statements that are subsequently rejected or weakened by the author. Furthermore, you should always read through the **entire passage** before drawing conclusions. Many readers are trained to expect the author's conclusions at either the beginning or the end of the passage, but many texts do not adhere to this format.

Identifying a logical conclusion can help you determine whether you agree with the writer or not. Coming to this conclusion is much like making an inference: the approach requires you to combine the information given by the text with what you already know in order to make a **logical conclusion**. If the author intended the reader to draw a certain conclusion, then you can expect the author's argumentation and detail to be leading in that direction. One way to approach the task of drawing conclusions is to make brief **notes** of all the points made by the author. When the notes are arranged on paper, they may clarify the logical conclusion. Another way to approach conclusions is to consider whether the reasoning of the author raises any **pertinent questions**. Sometimes you will be able to draw several conclusions from a passage. On occasion these will be conclusions that were never imagined by the author. Therefore, be aware that these conclusions must be **supported** directly by the text.

While being tested on your ability to make correct inferences, you must look for **contextual clues**. An answer can be *true* but not *correct*. The contextual clues will help you find the answer that is the **best answer** out of the given choices. Be careful in your reading to understand the context in which a phrase is stated. When asked for the implied meaning of a statement made in the passage, you should immediately locate the statement and read the **context** in which the statement was made. Also, look for an answer choice that has a similar phrase to the statement in question.

Readers are often required to understand a text that claims and suggests ideas without stating them directly. An **inference** is a piece of information that is implied but not written outright by the author. For instance, consider the following sentence: *After the final out of the inning, the fans were filled with joy and rushed the field*. From this sentence, a reader can infer that the fans were watching a baseball game and their team won the game. Readers should take great care to avoid using information **beyond the provided passage** before making inferences. As you practice drawing inferences, you will find that they require concentration and attention.

Describe the process of drawing conclusions.

Compare and contrast topics and main ideas.

Discuss the identification and evaluation of supporting details.

Visit *mometrix.com/academy* for a related video.
Enter video code: 396297

Discuss the use of topic and summary sentences.

Visit *mometrix.com/academy* for a related video.
Enter video code: 407801

Describe how to follow a given set of directions.

Describe the information to be found in a memo.

One of the most important skills in reading comprehension is the identification of **topics** and **main ideas.** There is a subtle difference between these two features. The topic is the **subject** of a text (i.e., what the text is all about). The main idea, on the other hand, is the **most important point** being made by the author. The topic is usually expressed in a few words at the most while the main idea often needs a full sentence to be completely defined. As an example, a short passage might have the topic of penguins and the main idea could be written as *Penguins are different from other birds in many ways*. In most nonfiction writing, the topic and the main idea will be stated directly and often appear in a sentence at the very beginning or end of the text. When being tested on an understanding of the author's topic, you may be able to skim the passage for the general idea, by reading only the first sentence of each paragraph. A body paragraph's first sentence is often—but not always—the main topic sentence which gives you a summary of the content in the paragraph.

However, there are cases in which the reader must figure out an **unstated** topic or main idea. In these instances, you must read every sentence of the text and try to come up with an overarching idea that is supported by each of those sentences.

Topic and summary sentences are a convenient way to encapsulate the **main idea** of a text. In some textbooks and academic articles, the author will place a **topic** or **summary sentence** at the beginning of each section as a means of preparing the reader for what is to come. Research suggests that the brain is more receptive to new information when it has been prepared by the presentation of the main idea or some key words. The phenomenon is somewhat akin to the primer coat of paint that allows subsequent coats of paint to absorb more easily. A good topic sentence will be **clear** and not contain any **jargon**. When topic or summary sentences are not provided, good readers can jot down their own so that they can find their place in a text and refresh their memory.

A memo (short for *memorandum*) is a common form of written communication. There is a standard format for these documents. It is typical for there to be a **heading** at the top indicating the author, date, and recipient. In some cases, this heading will also include the author's title and the name of his or her institution. Below this information will be the **body** of the memo. These documents are typically written by and for members of the same organization. They usually contain a plan of action, a request for information on a specific topic, or a response to such a request. Memos are considered to be official documents, and so are usually written in a **formal** style. Many memos are organized with numbers or bullet points, which make it easier for the reader to identify key ideas.

Drawing conclusions from information implied within a passage requires confidence on the part of the reader. **Implications** are things that the author does not state directly, but readers can assume based on what the author does say. Consider the following passage: *I stepped outside and opened my umbrella. By the time I got to work, the cuffs of my pants were soaked*. The author never states that it is raining, but this fact is clearly implied. Conclusions based on implication must be well supported by the text. In order to draw a solid conclusion, readers should have multiple pieces of **evidence**. If readers have only one piece, they must be assured that there is no other possible explanation than their conclusion. A good reader will be able to draw many conclusions from information implied by the text which will be a great help in the exam.

Supporting details provide **evidence** and backing for the main point. In order to show that a main idea is correct, or valid, authors add details that prove their point. All texts contain details, but they are only classified as **supporting details** when they serve to reinforce some larger point. Supporting details are most commonly found in **informative** and **persuasive** texts. In some cases, they will be clearly indicated with terms like *for example* or *for instance*, or they will be enumerated with terms like *first*, *second*, and *last*. However, you need to be prepared for texts that do not contain those indicators. As a reader, you should consider whether the author's supporting details really back up his or her **main point**. Supporting details can be factual and correct, yet they may not be relevant to the author's point. Conversely, supporting details can seem pertinent, but they can be ineffective because they are based on opinion or assertions that cannot be proven.

Technical passages often require the reader to **follow a set of directions**. For many people, especially those who are tactile or visual learners, this can be a difficult process. It is important to approach a set of directions differently than other texts. First, it is a good idea to **scan** the directions to determine whether special equipment or preparations are needed. Sometimes in a recipe, for instance, the author fails to mention that the oven should be preheated first, and then halfway through the process, the cook is supposed to be baking. After briefly reading the directions, the reader should return to the first step. When following directions, it is appropriate to **complete each step** before moving on to the next. If this is not possible, it is useful at least to visualize each step before reading the next.

Reading – Key Ideas and Details
© Mometrix Media - flashcardsecrets.com/teas
ATI TEAS Exam

Describe the information to be found in a posted announcement.

Reading – Key Ideas and Details
© Mometrix Media - flashcardsecrets.com/teas
ATI TEAS Exam

Describe the information to be found in a classified advertisement.

Reading – Key Ideas and Details
© Mometrix Media - flashcardsecrets.com/teas
ATI TEAS Exam

Describe how to identify scale readings when given a picture of a standard measurement instrument.

Reading – Key Ideas and Details
© Mometrix Media - flashcardsecrets.com/teas
ATI TEAS Exam

Describe how to use the legend or key of a map to identify specified information.

Reading – Key Ideas and Details
© Mometrix Media - flashcardsecrets.com/teas
ATI TEAS Exam

Describe how to identify a sequence in writing.

Visit *mometrix.com/academy* for a related video.
Enter video code: 489027

Reading – Craft and Structure
© Mometrix Media - flashcardsecrets.com/teas
ATI TEAS Exam

Describe some strategies for distinguishing between fact and opinion.

Visit *mometrix.com/academy* for related videos.
Enter video codes: 717670 and 870899

Classified advertisements, or **ads**, are used to sell or buy goods, to attract business, to make romantic connections, and to do countless other things. They are an inexpensive, and sometimes free, way to make a brief *pitch*. Classified ads used to be found only in newspapers or special advertising circulars, but there are now online listings as well. The style of these ads has remained basically the same. An ad usually begins with a word or phrase indicating what is being **sold** or **sought**. Then, the listing will give a brief **description** of the product or service. Because space is limited and costly in newspapers, classified ads there will often contain abbreviations for common attributes. For instance, two common abbreviations are *bk* for *black*, and *obo* for *or best offer*. Classified ads will then usually conclude by listing the **price** (or the amount the seeker is willing to pay), followed by **contact information** like a telephone number or email address.

People post **announcements** for all sorts of occasions. Many people are familiar with notices for lost pets, yard sales, and landscaping services. In order to be effective, these announcements need to *contain all of the information* the reader requires to act on the message. For instance, a lost pet announcement needs to include a good description of the animal and a contact number for the owner. A yard sale notice should include the address, date, and hours of the sale, as well as a brief description of the products that will be available there. When composing an announcement, it is important to consider the perspective of the **audience**—what will they need to know in order to respond to the message? Although a posted announcement can have color and decoration to attract the eye of the passerby, it must also convey the necessary information clearly.

Almost all maps contain a **key**, or **legend**, that defines the **symbols** used on the map for various landmarks. This key is usually placed in a corner of the map. It should contain listings for all of the important symbols on the map. Of course, these symbols will vary depending on the nature of the map. A road map uses different colored lines to indicate roads, highways, and interstates. A legend might also show different dots and squares that are used to indicate towns of various sizes. The legend may contain information about the map's **scale**, though this may be elsewhere on the map. Many legends will contain special symbols, such as a picnic table indicating a campground.

The scales used on **standard measurement instruments** are fairly easy to read with a little practice. Take the **ruler** as an example. A typical ruler has different units along each long edge. One side measures inches, and the other measures centimeters. The units are specified close to the zero reading for the ruler. Note that the ruler does not begin measuring from its outermost edge. The zero reading is a black line a tiny distance inside of the edge. On the inches side, each inch is indicated with a long black line and a number. Each half-inch is noted with a slightly shorter line. Quarter-inches are noted with still shorter lines, eighth-inches are noted with even shorter lines, and sixteenth-inches are noted with the shortest lines of all. On the centimeter side, the second-largest black lines indicate half-centimeters, and the smaller lines indicate tenths of centimeters, otherwise known as millimeters.

Readers must always be conscious of the distinction between **fact** and **opinion**. A fact can be subjected to analysis and can be either **proved or disproved**. An opinion, on the other hand, is the author's **personal thoughts or feelings** which may not be alterable by research or evidence. If the author writes that the distance from New York to Boston is about two hundred miles, then he or she is stating a fact. If the author writes that New York is too crowded, then he or she is giving an opinion because there is no objective standard for overpopulation.

An opinion may be indicated by words like *believe*, *think*, or *feel*. Readers must be aware that an **opinion** may be supported by **facts**. For instance, the author might give the population density of New York as evidence of an overcrowded population. An opinion supported by fact tends to be more convincing. On the other hand, when authors support their opinions with other opinions, readers should not be persuaded by the argument to any degree.

Readers must be able to identify a text's **sequence**, or the order in which things happen. Often, when the sequence is very important to the author, the text is indicated with signal words like *first*, *then*, *next*, and *last*. However, a sequence can be merely implied and must be noted by the reader. Consider the sentence: *He walked through the garden and gave water and fertilizer to the plants*. Clearly, the man did not walk through the garden before he collected water and fertilizer for the plants. So, the implied sequence is that he first collected water, then he collected fertilizer, next he walked through the garden, and last he gave water or fertilizer as necessary to the plants. Texts do not always proceed in an **orderly** sequence from first to last. Sometimes they begin at the end and start over at the beginning. As a reader, you can enhance your understanding of the passage by taking brief **notes** to clarify the sequence.

Reading – Craft and Structure
© Mometrix Media - flashcardsecrets.com/teas
ATI TEAS Exam

Discuss the identification of an author's biases and stereotypes.

Visit *mometrix.com/academy* for a related video.
Enter video code: 644829

Reading – Craft and Structure
© Mometrix Media - flashcardsecrets.com/teas
ATI TEAS Exam

Describe the problem-solution text structure.

Reading – Craft and Structure
© Mometrix Media - flashcardsecrets.com/teas
ATI TEAS Exam

Explain what a descriptive text is.

Visit *mometrix.com/academy* for a related video.
Enter video code: 174903

Reading – Craft and Structure
© Mometrix Media - flashcardsecrets.com/teas
ATI TEAS Exam

Describe how an author compares and contrasts.

Visit *mometrix.com/academy* for a related video.
Enter video code: 171799

Reading – Craft and Structure
© Mometrix Media - flashcardsecrets.com/teas
ATI TEAS Exam

Describe how an author demonstrates cause and effect.

Visit *mometrix.com/academy* for a related video.
Enter video code: 725944

Reading – Craft and Structure
© Mometrix Media - flashcardsecrets.com/teas
ATI TEAS Exam

Describe the characteristics of a narrative passage.

Some nonfiction texts are organized to present a **problem** followed by a **solution**. For this type of text, the problem is often explained before the solution is offered. In some cases, as when the problem is well known, the solution may be introduced briefly at the beginning. Other passages may focus on the solution, and the problem will be referenced only occasionally. Some texts will outline *multiple solutions* to a problem, leaving readers to choose among them. If the author has an interest or an allegiance to one solution, he or she may fail to mention or describe accurately some of the other solutions. Readers should be careful of the author's **agenda** when reading a problem-solution text. Only by understanding the author's perspective and interests can one develop a proper judgment of the proposed solution.

Every author has a point-of-view, but authors demonstrate a **bias** when they ignore reasonable counterarguments or distort opposing viewpoints. A bias is evident whenever the author is **unfair** or **inaccurate** in his or her presentation. Bias may be intentional or unintentional, and readers should be skeptical of the author's argument. Remember that a biased author may still be correct; however, the author will be correct in spite of his or her bias, not because of the bias. A **stereotype** is like a bias, yet a stereotype is applied specifically to a **group** or **place**. Stereotyping is considered to be particularly abhorrent because the practice promotes negative generalizations about people. Readers should be very cautious of authors who stereotype in their writing. These faulty assumptions typically reveal the author's ignorance and lack of curiosity.

Authors will use different stylistic and writing devices to make their meaning clear for readers. One of those devices is **comparison and contrast**. As mentioned previously, when an author describes the ways in which two things are **alike**, he or she is comparing them. When the author describes the ways in which two things are **different**, he or she is contrasting them. The "compare and contrast" essay is one of the most common forms in nonfiction. These passages are often signaled with certain words: a comparison may have indicating terms such as *both*, *same*, *like*, *too*, and *as well*; while a contrast may have terms like *but*, *however*, *on the other hand*, *instead*, and *yet*. Of course, comparisons and contrasts may be implicit without using any such signaling language. A single sentence may both compare and contrast. Consider the sentence *Brian and Sheila love ice cream, but Brian prefers vanilla and Sheila prefers strawberry*. In one sentence, the author has described both a similarity (love of ice cream) and a difference (favorite flavor).

In a sense, almost all writing is descriptive, insofar as an author seeks to describe events, ideas, or people to the reader. Some texts, however, are primarily concerned with **description**. A descriptive text focuses on a particular subject and attempts to depict the subject in a way that will be clear to readers. Descriptive texts contain many adjectives and adverbs (i.e., words that give shades of meaning and create a more detailed mental picture for the reader). A descriptive text fails when it is unclear to the reader. A descriptive text will certainly be informative and may be persuasive and entertaining as well.

A **narrative** passage is a story that can be fiction or nonfiction. However, there are a few elements that a text must have in order to be classified as a narrative. First, the text must have a **plot** (i.e., a series of events). Narratives often proceed in a clear sequence, but this is not a requirement. If the narrative is good, then these events will be interesting to readers. Second, a narrative has **characters**. These characters could be people, animals, or even inanimate objects—so long as they participate in the plot. Third, a narrative passage often contains **figurative language** which is meant to stimulate the imagination of readers by making comparisons and observations. For instance, a *metaphor*, a common piece of figurative language, is a description of one thing in terms of another. *The moon was a frosty snowball* is an example of a metaphor. In the literal sense this is obviously untrue, but the comparison suggests a certain mood for the reader.

One of the most common text structures is **cause and effect**. A cause is an **act** or **event** that makes something happen, and an effect is the thing that happens as a **result** of the cause. A cause-and-effect relationship is not always explicit, but there are some terms in English that signal causes, such as *since*, *because*, and *due to*. Furthermore, terms that signal effects include *consequently*, *therefore*, *this lead(s) to*. As an example, consider this sentence: *Because the sky was clear, Ron did not bring an umbrella*. The cause is the clear sky, and the effect is that Ron did not bring an umbrella. However, readers may find that sometimes the cause-and-effect relationship will not be clearly noted. For instance, the sentence *He was late and missed the meeting* does not contain any signaling words, but the sentence still contains a cause (he was late) and an effect (he missed the meeting).

Reading – Craft and Structure
© Mometrix Media - flashcardsecrets.com/teas
ATI TEAS Exam

Describe the characteristics of an expository passage.

Reading – Craft and Structure
© Mometrix Media - flashcardsecrets.com/teas
ATI TEAS Exam

Describe the characteristics of a technical passage.

Reading – Craft and Structure
© Mometrix Media - flashcardsecrets.com/teas
ATI TEAS Exam

Describe the characteristics of a persuasive passage.

Reading – Craft and Structure
© Mometrix Media - flashcardsecrets.com/teas
ATI TEAS Exam

Describe how to identify the correct definition of a word when given the word in context.

Reading – Craft and Structure
© Mometrix Media - flashcardsecrets.com/teas
ATI TEAS Exam

Describe the different types of language authors use to convey meaning.

Reading – Craft and Structure
© Mometrix Media - flashcardsecrets.com/teas
ATI TEAS Exam

Describe what a metaphor is.

Visit *mometrix.com/academy* for a related video.
Enter video code: 133295

A **technical** passage is written to *describe* a complex object or process. Technical writing is common in medical and technological fields, in which complex ideas of mathematics, science, and engineering need to be explained *simply* and *clearly*. To ease comprehension, a technical passage usually proceeds in a very logical order. Technical passages often have clear headings and subheadings, which are used to keep the reader oriented in the text. Additionally, you will find that these passages divide sections up with numbers or letters. Many technical passages look more like an outline than a piece of prose. The amount of **jargon** or difficult vocabulary will vary in a technical passage depending on the intended audience. As much as possible, technical passages try to avoid language that the reader will have to research in order to understand the message, yet readers will find that jargon cannot always be avoided.

An **expository** passage aims to **inform** and enlighten readers. The passage is nonfiction and usually centers around a simple, easily defined topic. Since the goal of exposition is to teach, such a passage should be as clear as possible. Often, an expository passage contains helpful organizing words, like *first*, *next*, *for example*, and *therefore*. These words keep the reader **oriented** in the text. Although expository passages do not need to feature colorful language and artful writing, they are often more effective with these features. For a reader, the challenge of expository passages is to maintain steady attention. Expository passages are not always about subjects that will naturally interest a reader, so the writer is often more concerned with **clarity** and **comprehensibility** than with engaging the reader. By reading actively, you will ensure a good habit of focus when reading an expository passage.

One of the benefits of reading is the expansion of one's vocabulary. In order to obtain this benefit, however, one needs to know how to identify the definition of a **word from its context**. This means defining a word based on the **words around it** and the way it is **used in a sentence**. Consider the following sentence: *The elderly scholar spent his evenings hunched over arcane texts that few other people even knew existed.* The adjective *arcane* is uncommon, but you can obtain significant information about it based on its use in the sentence. The fact that few other people know of their existence allows you to assume that "arcane texts" must be rare and be of interest to few people. Also, the texts are being read by an elderly scholar. So, you can assume that they focus on difficult academic subjects. Sometimes, words can be defined by **what they are not**. Consider the following sentence: *Ron's fealty to his parents was not shared by Karen, who disobeyed their every command.* Someone who disobeys is not demonstrating *fealty*. So, you can infer that the word means something like *obedience* or *respect*.

A **persuasive** passage is meant to change the mind of readers and lead them into **agreement** with the author. The persuasive intent may be very obvious or quite difficult to discern. In some cases, a persuasive passage will be indistinguishable from one that is informative. Both passages make an assertion and offer supporting details. However, a persuasive passage is more likely to appeal to the reader's **emotions** and to make claims based on **opinion**. Persuasive passages may not describe alternate positions, but when they do, they often display significant **bias**. Readers may find that a persuasive passage is giving the author's viewpoint, or the passage may adopt a seemingly objective tone. A persuasive passage is successful if it can make a convincing argument and win the trust of the reader.

A **metaphor** is a type of figurative language in which the writer equates one thing with a different thing. For instance: *The bird was an arrow arcing through the sky*. In this sentence, the arrow is serving as a metaphor for the bird. The point of a metaphor is to encourage the reader to consider the item being described in a *different way*. Let's continue with this metaphor for a bird: you are asked to envision the bird's flight as being similar to the arc of an arrow. So, you imagine the flight to be swift and bending. Metaphors are a way for the author to describe an item *without being direct and obvious*. This literary device is a lyrical and suggestive way of providing information. Note that the reference for a metaphor will not always be mentioned explicitly by the author. Consider the following description of a forest in winter: *Swaying skeletons reached for the sky and groaned as the wind blew through them.* In this example, the author is using *skeletons* as a metaphor for leafless trees. This metaphor creates a spooky tone while inspiring the reader's imagination.

There are many types of language devices that authors use to convey their meaning in a descriptive way. Understanding these concepts will help you understand what you read. These types of devices are called **figurative language** – language that goes beyond the literal meaning of a word or phrase. **Descriptive language** that evokes imagery in the reader's mind is one type of figurative language. **Exaggeration** is another type of figurative language. Also, when you compare two things, you are using figurative language. **Similes** and **metaphors** are ways of comparing things, and both are types of figurative language commonly found in poetry. An example of figurative language (a simile in this case): *The child howled like a coyote when her mother told her to pick up the toys.* In this example, the child's howling is compared to that of a coyote and helps the reader understand the sound being made by the child.

Describe what a simile is.

Describe what personification is.

Describe the difference between denotative and connotative meaning.

Describe how to identify the correct definition of a word when given a sample entry in which the definition of the word may be found.

Discuss the issues related to identifying an author's purpose.

Describe some strategies for identifying an author's purpose.

Another type of figurative language is **personification**. This is the description of a nonhuman thing as if the item were **human**. Literally, the word means the process of making something into a person. The general intent of personification is to describe things in a manner that will be comprehensible to readers. When an author states that a tree *groans* in the wind, he or she does not mean that the tree is emitting a low, pained sound from a mouth. Instead, the author means that the tree is making a noise similar to a human groan. Of course, this personification establishes a tone of sadness or suffering. A different tone would be established if the author said that the tree was *swaying* or *dancing*.

A **simile** is a figurative expression that is similar to a metaphor, yet the expression requires the use of the distancing words *like* or *as*. Some examples: *The sun was like an orange, eager as a beaver*, and *nimble as a mountain goat*. Because a simile includes *like* or *as*, the device creates a space between the description and the thing being described. If an author says that *a house was like a shoebox*, then the tone is different than the author saying that the house *was* a shoebox. In a simile, authors explicitly indicate that the description is **not** the same thing as the thing being described. In a metaphor, there is no such distinction. The decision of which device to use will be made based on the authors' intended **tone**.

Dictionaries can be used to find a word's meaning, to check spelling, and to find out how to say or pronounce a word. **Dictionary entries** are in alphabetical order. **Guide words** are the two words at the top of each page. One word is the first word listed on the page and the other word is the last word listed on the page. Using these guide words will help you use the dictionaries more effectively. You may notice that many words have more than one definition. These different definitions are numbered. Also, some words can be used as different **parts of speech**. The definitions for each part of speech are separated. A simple entry might look like this:

WELL: (adverb) 1. in a good way | (noun) 1. a hole drilled into the earth
The correct definition of a word depends on how the word is used in a sentence. To know that you are using the word correctly, you can try to replace the dictionary's definitions for the word in the passage. Then, choose the definition that seems to be the best fit.

The **denotative** meaning of a word is the literal meaning of the word. The **connotative** meaning goes beyond the denotative meaning to include the **emotional reaction** that a word may invoke. The connotative meaning often takes the denotative meaning a step further due to associations which the reader makes with the denotative meaning. Readers can differentiate between the denotative and connotative meanings by first recognizing how authors use each meaning. Most nonfiction, for example, is fact-based and authors do not use flowery, figurative language. The reader can assume that the writer is using the denotative meaning of words. In fiction, the author may use the connotative meaning. Readers can determine whether the author is using the denotative or connotative meaning of a word by implementing **context clues**.

An author's purpose is evident often in the **organization** of the text (e.g., section headings in bold font points to an informative text). However, you may not have such organization available to you in your exam. Instead, if the author makes his or her main idea clear from the beginning, then the likely purpose of the text is to **inform**. If the author begins by making a claim and provides various arguments to support that claim, then the purpose is probably to **persuade**. If the author tells a story or seems to want the attention of the reader more than to push a particular point or deliver information, then his or her purpose is most likely to **entertain**. As a reader, you must judge authors on how well they accomplish their purpose. In other words, you need to consider the type of passage (e.g., technical, persuasive, etc.) that the author has written and whether the author has followed the requirements of the passage type.

Usually, identifying the **purpose** of an author is easier than identifying his or her position. In most cases, the author has no interest in hiding his or her purpose. A text that is meant to entertain, for instance, should be written to please the reader. Most narratives, or stories, are written to entertain, though they may also inform or persuade. Informative texts are easy to identify, while the most difficult purpose of a text to identify is persuasion because the author has an interest in making this purpose hard to detect. When a reader discovers that the author is trying to persuade, he or she should be skeptical of the argument. For this reason, persuasive texts often try to establish an entertaining tone and hope to amuse the reader into agreement. On the other hand, an informative tone may be implemented to create an appearance of authority and objectivity.

Discuss the identification of the author's intent to persuade.

Discuss the identification of the author's intent to inform.

Visit *mometrix.com/academy* for a related video.
Enter video code: 924964

Discuss the identification of the author's intent to entertain.

Discuss the identification of the author's intent to express feelings.

Discuss some strategies for identifying an author's position.

Analyze the use of headings and subheadings.

An **informative text** is written to educate and enlighten readers. Informative texts are almost always nonfiction and are rarely structured as a story. The intention of an informative text is to deliver information in the most comprehensible way. So, look for the structure of the text to be very clear. In an informative text, the thesis statement is one or two sentences that normally appears at the end of the first paragraph. The author may use some colorful language, but he or she is likely to put more emphasis on clarity and precision. Informative essays do not typically appeal to the emotions. They often contain facts and figures and rarely include the opinion of the author; however, readers should remain aware of the possibility for a bias as those facts are presented. Sometimes a persuasive essay can resemble an informative essay, especially if the author maintains an even tone and presents his or her views as if they were established fact.

In a persuasive essay, the author is attempting to change the reader's mind or **convince** him or her of something that he or she did not believe previously. There are several identifying characteristics of **persuasive writing**. One is **opinion presented as fact**. When authors attempt to persuade readers, they often present their opinions as if they were fact. Readers must be on guard for statements that sound factual but which cannot be subjected to research, observation, or experiment. Another characteristic of persuasive writing is **emotional language**. An author will often try to play on the emotions of readers by appealing to their sympathy or sense of morality. When an author uses colorful or evocative language with the intent of arousing the reader's passions, then the author may be attempting to persuade. Finally, in many cases, a persuasive text will give an **unfair explanation of opposing positions**, if these positions are mentioned at all.

When an author intends to **express feelings,** he or she may use **expressive and bold language**. An author may write with emotion for any number of reasons. Sometimes, authors will express feelings because they are describing a personal situation of great pain or happiness. In other situations, authors will attempt to persuade the reader and will use emotion to stir up the passions. This kind of expression is easy to identify when the writer uses phrases like *I felt* and *I sense*. However, readers may find that the author will simply describe feelings without introducing them. As a reader, you must know the importance of recognizing when an author is expressing emotion and not to become overwhelmed by sympathy or passion. Readers should maintain some **detachment** so that they can still evaluate the strength of the author's argument or the quality of the writing.

The success or failure of an author's intent to **entertain** is determined by those who read the author's work. Entertaining texts may be either fiction or nonfiction, and they may describe real or imagined people, places, and events. Entertaining texts are often narratives or poems. A text that is written to entertain is likely to contain **colorful language** that engages the imagination and the emotions. Such writing often features a great deal of figurative language, which typically enlivens the subject matter with images and analogies.

Though an entertaining text is not usually written to persuade or inform, authors may accomplish both of these tasks in their work. An entertaining text may *appeal to the reader's emotions* and cause him or her to think differently about a particular subject. In any case, entertaining texts tend to showcase the personality of the author more than other types of writing.

Many informative texts, especially textbooks, use **headings** and **subheadings** for organization. Headings and subheadings are printed in larger and bolder fonts than the rest of the text. Sometimes, they are in a different color than the main body of the book. Headings are often larger than subheadings. Also, headings and subheadings are not always complete sentences. A heading gives the **topic** that will be addressed in the paragraphs below. Headings are meant to alert you about what is coming next. Subheadings give the **topics of smaller sections**. For example, the heading of a section in a science textbook might be *AMPHIBIANS*. Within that section, you may have subheadings for *Frogs*, *Salamanders*, and *Newts*. Pay close attention to headings and subheadings. They make it easy to go back and find specific details in a book.

In order to be an effective reader, one must pay attention to the author's **position** and purpose. Even those texts that seem objective and impartial, like textbooks, have a position and **bias**. Readers need to take these positions into account when considering the author's message. When an author uses emotional language or clearly favors one side of an argument, his or her position is clear. However, the author's position may be evident not only in what he or she writes, but also in what he or she doesn't write. In a normal setting, a reader would want to review some other texts on the same topic in order to develop a view of the author's position. If this was not possible, then you would want to acquire some *background* about the author. However, since you are in the middle of an exam and the only source of information is the text, you should look for *language and argumentation that seems to indicate a particular stance* on the subject.

Reading – Craft and Structure

Describe the use of footnotes.

Reading – Craft and Structure

Describe the use of bold text and underlining.

Reading – Craft and Structure

Describe the use of italics in a text.

Reading – Craft and Structure

Explain how to obtain information from an index.

Reading – Craft and Structure

Explain how to obtain information from a table of contents.

Reading – Integration of Knowledge and Ideas

Explain the process of identifying appropriate primary sources.

Authors will often incorporate text features like bold text and underlining to communicate meaning to the reader. When text is made **bold**, it is often because the author wants to emphasize the point that is being made. Bold text indicates **importance**. Also, many textbooks place key terms in bold. This not only draws the reader's attention, but also makes it easy to find these terms when reviewing before a test. **Underlining** serves a similar purpose. It is often used to suggest **emphasis**. However, underlining is also used on occasion beneath the **titles** of books, magazines, and works of art. This was more common when people used typewriters, which weren't able to create italics. Now that word processing software is nearly universal, italics are generally used for longer works.

Footnotes and endnotes can also be used in word processing programs. A **footnote** is text that is listed at the *bottom of a page* which lists where facts and figures within that document page were obtained. An **endnote** is similar to a footnote, but differs in the fact that it is listed at the *end of paragraphs and chapters* of a document, instead of the bottom of each page of the document.

Normally, a nonfiction book will have an **index** at the end. The index is for you to find information about specific topics. An index lists the topics in alphabetical order (i.e., a, b, c, d...). The names of people are listed by last name. For example, *Adams, John* would come before *Washington, George*. To the right of a topic, the page numbers are listed for that topic. When a topic is spread over several pages, the index will connect these pages with a dash. For example, if a topic is said to be on pages 35 to 42 and again on 53, the topic will be labeled as 35–42, 53. Some topics will have **subtopics**. These subtopics are listed below the main topic, indented slightly, and placed in alphabetical order. This is common for subjects that are covered over several pages in the book. For example, if you have a book about Elizabethan drama, William Shakespeare is likely an important topic. Beneath Shakespeare's name in the index, you may find listings for *death of, dramatic works of, life of,* etc. These specific subtopics help you narrow your search.

Italics, like bold text and underlines, are used to **emphasize** important words, phrases, and sentences in a text. However, italics have other uses as well. A word is placed in italics when it is being discussed *as* a word; that is, when it is being **defined** or its use in a sentence is being **described**. For instance, it is appropriate to use italics when saying that *esoteric* is an unusual adjective. Italics are also used for the titles of long or large works, like books, magazines, long operas, and epic poems. Shorter works are typically placed within **quotation marks**. A reader should note how an author uses italics, as this is a marker of *style and tone*. Some authors use them frequently, creating a tone of high emotion, while others are more restrained in their use, suggesting calm and reason.

When conducting research, it is important to depend on reputable **primary sources**. A primary source is the **documentary evidence** closest to the subject being studied. For instance, the primary sources for an essay about penguins would be photographs and recordings of the birds, as well as accounts of people who have studied penguins in person. A **secondary source** would be a review of a movie about penguins or a book outlining the observations made by others. A primary source should be credible and, if it is on a subject that is still being explored, recent. One way to assess the credibility of a work is to see how often it is mentioned in other books and articles on the same subject. Just by reading the works cited and bibliographies of other books, one can get a sense of what the reliable sources authorities in the field are.

Most books, magazines, and journals have a **table of contents** at the beginning. The table of contents lists the different **subjects** or **chapter titles** with a page number. This information allows you to find what you need with ease. Normally, the table of contents is found a page or two after the title page in a book or in the first few pages of a magazine. In a book, the table of contents will have the chapters listed on the left side. The page number for each chapter comes on the right side. Many books have a **preface** (i.e., a note that explains the background of the book) or introduction. The preface and introduction come with Roman numerals. The chapters are listed in order from the beginning to the end.

Reading – Integration of Knowledge and Ideas

Explain the process of identifying appropriate Internet sources.

Reading – Integration of Knowledge and Ideas

Discuss the use of prior knowledge to make predictions about a piece of literature.

Visit *mometrix.com/academy* for a related video.
Enter video code: 437248

Reading – Integration of Knowledge and Ideas

Describe the use of foreshadowing.

Reading – Integration of Knowledge and Ideas

Discuss drawing conclusions and the importance of answering the related questions only from the reading.

Reading – Integration of Knowledge and Ideas

Discuss the identification and evaluation of themes.

Visit *mometrix.com/academy* for a related video.
Enter video code: 732074

Reading – Integration of Knowledge and Ideas

Discuss how literature from different cultures presents similar themes.

A prediction is a **guess** about what will happen next. Readers constantly make predictions based on what they have read and what they already know. Consider the following sentence: *Staring at the computer screen in shock, Kim blindly reached over for the brimming glass of water on the shelf to her side.* The sentence suggests that Kim is agitated, and that she is not looking at the glass that she is going to pick up. So, a reader might **predict** that Kim is going to knock over the glass. Of course, not every prediction will be accurate: perhaps Kim will pick the glass up cleanly. Nevertheless, the author has certainly created the expectation that the water might be spilled. Predictions are always subject to revision as the reader acquires more information.

The Internet was once considered a poor place to find sources for an essay or article, but its credibility has improved greatly over the years. Still, students need to exercise caution when performing research online. The best sources are those affiliated with **established institutions**, such as *universities, public libraries, and think tanks*. Most newspapers are available online, and many of them allow the public to browse their archives. Magazines frequently offer similar services. When obtaining information from an unknown website, however, one must exercise considerably more caution. A website can be considered trustworthy if it is referenced by other sites that are known to be reputable. Also, credible sites tend to be properly maintained and frequently updated. A site is easier to trust when the author provides some information about himself, including some credentials that indicate expertise in the subject matter.

In addition to inference and prediction, readers must often **draw conclusions** about the information they have read. When asked for a *conclusion* that may be drawn, look for critical "hedge" phrases, such as *likely, may, can, will often*, among many others. When you are being tested on this knowledge, remember the question that writers insert into these hedge phrases to cover every possibility. Often an answer will be wrong simply because there is no room for exception. Extreme positive or negative answers (such as always or never) are usually not correct. The reader should not use any outside knowledge that is not gathered from the passage to answer the related questions. Correct answers can be derived *straight from the passage*.

Foreshadowing uses hints in a narrative to let the audience **anticipate** future events in the plot. Foreshadowing can be indicated by a number of literary devices and figures of speech, as well as through dialogue between characters.

A brief study of world literature suggests that writers from vastly different cultures address **similar themes**. For instance, works like the *Odyssey* and *Hamlet* both consider the individual's battle for self-control and independence. In most cultures, authors address themes of *personal growth and the struggle for maturity*. Another universal theme is the *conflict between the individual and society*. Works that are as culturally disparate as *Native Son*, the *Aeneid*, and *1984* dramatize how people struggle to maintain their personalities and dignity in large (sometimes) oppressive groups. Finally, many cultures have versions of the *hero's or heroine's journey* in which an adventurous person must overcome many obstacles in order to gain greater knowledge, power, and perspective. Some famous works that treat this theme are the *Epic of Gilgamesh*, Dante's *Divine Comedy*, and Cervantes' *Don Quixote*.

Themes are seldom expressed directly in a text and can be difficult to identify. A **theme** is *an issue, an idea, or a question raised by the text*. For instance, a theme of *Cinderella* (the Charles Perrault version) is perseverance as the title character serves her step-sisters and step-mother, and the prince seeks to find the girl with the missing slipper. A passage may have many themes, and you, as a dedicated reader, must take care to identify only themes that you are asked to find. One common characteristic of themes is that they raise more questions than they answer. In a good piece of fiction, authors are trying to elevate the reader's perspective and encourage him or her to consider the themes in a deeper way. In the process of reading, one can identify themes by constantly *asking about the general issues that the text is addressing*. A good way to evaluate an author's approach to a theme is to begin reading with a question in mind (e.g., How does this text approach the theme of love?) and to look for evidence in the text that addresses that question.

Discuss how literature of various cultures and genres addresses themes differently.

Describe argumentative and persuasive passages.

Explain how text evidence helps lead the reader to a conclusion.

Describe credibility within a text.

Visit *mometrix.com/academy* for a related video.
Enter video code: 486236

Describe how an author may appeal to the reader's emotion.

Explain how an author builds trust with the reader.

Argumentative and persuasive passages take a **stand** on a debatable issue, seek to explore all sides of the issue, and find the best possible solution. Argumentative and persuasive passages should not be combative or abusive. The word *argument* may remind you of two or more people shouting at each other and walking away in anger. However, an argumentative or persuasive passage should be a *calm and reasonable presentation of an author's ideas* for others to consider. When an author writes reasonable arguments, his or her goal is not to win or have the last word. Instead, authors want to reveal current understanding of the question at hand and suggest a **solution** to a problem. The purpose of argument and persuasion in a free society is to reach the best solution.

Authors from different **genres** and **cultures** may address similar themes, but they do so in different ways. For instance, poets are likely to address subject matter indirectly through the use of *images and allusions*. In a play, the author is more likely to dramatize themes by using characters to express opposing viewpoints; this disparity is known as a *dialectical approach*. In a passage, the author does not need to express themes directly; indeed, they can be expressed through *events and actions*. In some regional literatures, such as Greece or England, authors use more irony: their works have characters that express views and make decisions that are clearly disapproved of by the author. In Latin America, there is a great tradition of using supernatural events to illustrate themes about real life. Chinese and Japanese authors frequently use well-established regional forms (e.g., haiku poetry in Japan) to organize their treatment of universal themes

The text used to support an argument can be the argument's downfall if the text is not credible. A text is **credible**, or believable, when the author is knowledgeable and objective, or unbiased. The author's **motivations** for writing the text play a critical role in determining the credibility of the text and must be evaluated when assessing that credibility. Reports written about the ozone layer by an environmental scientist and a hairdresser will have different levels of credibility.

The term **text evidence** refers to information that supports a **main point** or **minor points** and can help lead the reader to a conclusion. Information used as text evidence is precise, descriptive, and factual. A main point is often followed by **supporting details** that provide evidence to back up a claim. For example, a passage may include the claim that winter occurs during opposite months in the Northern and Southern hemispheres. Text evidence based on this claim may include countries where winter occurs in opposite months along with reasons that winter occurs at different times of the year in separate hemispheres (due to the tilt of the Earth as it rotates around the sun).

Evidence needs to be provided that supports the thesis and additional arguments. Most arguments must be supported by facts or statistics. A **fact** is something that is *known with certainty* and has been verified by several independent individuals. **Examples** and **illustrations** add an emotional component to arguments. With this component, you persuade readers in ways that facts and statistics cannot. The emotional component is effective when used with objective information that can be confirmed.

When authors give both sides to the argument, they build trust with their readers. As a reader, you should start with an undecided or neutral position. If an author presents only his or her side to the argument, then you will need to be concerned at best.

Building common ground with neutral or opposed readers can be appealing to skeptical readers. Sharing values with undecided readers can allow people to switch positions without giving up what they feel is important. For people who may oppose a position, they need to feel that they can change their minds without betraying who they are as a person. This *appeal to having an open mind* can be a powerful tool in arguing a position without antagonizing other views. Objections can be countered on a point-by-point basis or in a summary paragraph. Be mindful of how an author points out flaws in **counterarguments**. If they are unfair to the other side of the argument, then you should lose trust with the author.

Sometimes, authors will **appeal to the reader's emotion** in an attempt to *persuade or to distract the reader from the weakness of the argument*. For instance, the author may try to inspire the **pity** of the reader by delivering a heart-rending story. An author also might use the **bandwagon** approach, in which he suggests that his opinion is correct because it is held by the majority. Some authors resort to **name-calling**, in which insults and harsh words are delivered to the opponent in an attempt to distract. In advertising, a common appeal is the **celebrity testimonial**, in which a famous person endorses a product. Of course, the fact that a famous person likes something should not really mean anything to the reader. These and other emotional appeals are usually evidence of poor reasoning and a weak argument.

Reading – Integration of Knowledge and Ideas

Describe the criteria used to evaluate published journal articles.

Reading – Integration of Knowledge and Ideas

Describe the process of reading a line graph.

Reading – Integration of Knowledge and Ideas

Describe the process of reading a bar graph.

Reading – Integration of Knowledge and Ideas

Describe the process of reading a pie chart.

Reading – Integration of Knowledge and Ideas

Describe the different roles of library media specialists.

Reading – Integration of Knowledge and Ideas

Describe the function of an information specialist.

A line graph is a type of graph that is typically used for *measuring trends over time*. The graph is set up along a vertical and a horizontal **axis**. The variables being measured are listed along the left side and the bottom side of the axes. Points are then plotted along the graph as they correspond with their values for each variable. For instance, imagine a line graph measuring a person's income for each month of the year. If the person earned $1500 in January, there should be a point directly above January (perpendicular to the horizontal axis) and directly to the right of $1500 (perpendicular to the vertical axis). Once all of the lines are plotted, they are connected with a line from left to right. This line provides a nice visual illustration of the general **trends**. For instance, using the earlier example, if the line sloped up, then one would see that the person's income had increased over the course of the year.

Although published journal articles listed in library databases have been reviewed and edited to be acceptable for publication, you should still evaluate them by six criteria.

1. **Source**: Articles by experts in their subjects, published in scholarly journals, are more *reliable*. They also contain *references* to more publications on the same topic. Try to start your search with a database that includes searching by article type (e.g., reviews, clinical trials, editorials, and research articles).
2. **Length**: The citation states an article's number of pages, an indication of its research *utility*.
3. **Authority**: Research sources should be authoritative, written by *experts* affiliated with academic institutions.
4. **Date**: Many research fields are constantly changing, so research must be as *current* as possible. In areas with new research breakthroughs, some articles are not up-to-date.
5. **Audience**: If an author wrote an article for professional colleagues, it will include subject-specific language and *terminology*.
6. **Usefulness**: Evaluate whether an article is *relevant* to one's own research topic.

A pie chart, also known as a circle graph, is useful for depicting how a single unit or category is divided. The standard pie chart is a circle with designated wedges. Each wedge is **proportional** in size to a part of the whole. For instance, consider a pie chart representing a student's budget. If the student spends half of his or her money on rent, then the pie chart will represent that amount with a line through the center of the pie. If she spends a quarter of her money on food, there will be a line extending from the edge of the circle to the center at a right angle to the line depicting rent. This illustration would make it clear that the student spends twice the amount of money on rent as she does on food.

A pie chart is effective at showing how a single entity is *divided into parts*. They are not effective at demonstrating the relationships between parts of different wholes. For example, an unhelpful use of a pie chart would be to compare the respective amounts of state and federal spending devoted to infrastructure since these values are only meaningful in the context of the entire budget.

The bar graph is one of the most common visual representations of information. **Bar graphs** are used to illustrate sets of numerical **data**. The graph has a vertical axis (along which numbers are listed) and a horizontal axis (along which categories, words, or some other indicators are placed). One example of a bar graph is a depiction of the respective heights of famous basketball players: the vertical axis would contain numbers ranging from five to eight feet, and the horizontal axis would contain the names of the players. The length of the bar above the player's name would illustrate his height, and the top of the bar would stop perpendicular to the height listed along the left side. In this representation, one would see that Yao Ming is taller than Michael Jordan because Yao's bar would be higher.

In fulfilling the function of an **information specialist**, library media specialists bring their skills for finding and evaluating information in a variety of formats as resources for learners and educators. They bring an awareness of various issues related to information to the attention of students, teachers, administrators, and other involved parties. Library media specialists also serve to model for students the **strategies** they can learn to find, access, and evaluate information inside and outside of the library media centers. The environment of the library media center has experienced a critical impact from the development of technology. Accordingly, the library media specialist not only attains mastery over current advanced electronic resources, but she or he must also continually sustain attention focused on how information—both in more traditional forms and in the newest technological forms—is used ethically, as well as its quality and its character.

Today's **library media specialists** are important figures in contemporary learning communities, which now consist of administrators, teachers, and parents; and international, national, state, regional, and local communities. Such communities transcend the borders of disciplinary field, occupation, age, time, and place. They are connected by shared needs, interests, and rapidly increasing technologies in telecommunications. Library media specialists and student-centered library media programs aim to aid students in attaining and improving their **information literacy**. As such, library media specialists and library media programs have the objective of helping every student to creatively and actively find, evaluate, and use information toward the ends of fulfilling their own curiosities and imaginations by pursuing reading and research activities and of exercising and developing their own critical thinking abilities.

Reading – Integration of Knowledge and Ideas
© Mometrix Media - flashcardsecrets.com/teas
ATI TEAS Exam

Describe the process of organizing information for research.

Reading – Integration of Knowledge and Ideas
© Mometrix Media - flashcardsecrets.com/teas
ATI TEAS Exam

Describe the six major types of logical organization.

Reading – Integration of Knowledge and Ideas
© Mometrix Media - flashcardsecrets.com/teas
ATI TEAS Exam

Describe the process of generating questions about data you collected.

Mathematics – Numbers and Operations
© Mometrix Media - flashcardsecrets.com/teas
ATI TEAS Exam

Describe the different types of numbers.

Mathematics – Numbers and Operations
© Mometrix Media - flashcardsecrets.com/teas
ATI TEAS Exam

Describe the uses of decimals.

Mathematics – Numbers and Operations
© Mometrix Media - flashcardsecrets.com/teas
ATI TEAS Exam

Describe rational, irrational, and real numbers.

Visit *mometrix.com/academy* for related videos.
Enter video codes: 461071 and 280645

There are six major types of logical organization that are frequently used:
1. **Illustrations** may be used to support the thesis. Examples are the most common form of this organization.
2. **Definitions** say what something is or is not. A helpful question for this type of organization is, "What are the characteristics of the topic?"
3. Dividing or **classifying** information into separate items according to their similarities is a common and effective organizing method.
4. **Comparing** (focusing on the similarities of things) and contrasting (highlighting the differences between things) are excellent tools to use with certain kinds of information.
5. **Cause and effect** is a simple tool to logically understand relationships between things. A phenomenon may be traced to its causes for organizing a subject logically.
6. **Problem and solution** is a simple and effective manner of logically organizing material. It is very commonly used and lucidly presents information.

Organizing information effectively is an important part of research. The data must be organized in a useful manner so that it can be effectively used. Three basic ways to organize information are:
1. **Spatial Organization** – This is useful as it lets the user "see" the information, to fix it in *space*. This has benefits for those individuals who are visually adept at processing information.
2. **Chronological Organization** – This is the most common presentation of information. This method places information in the *sequence* with which it occurs. Chronological organization is very useful in explaining a process that occurs in a step-by-step pattern.
3. **Logical Organization** – This includes presenting material in a logical *pattern* that makes intuitive sense. Some patterns that are frequently used are illustrated, definition, compare/contrast, cause/effect, problem/solution, and division/classification.

Integer – any positive or negative whole number, including zero. Integers do not include fractions $\left(\frac{1}{3}\right)$, decimals (0.56), or mixed numbers $\left(7\frac{3}{4}\right)$.

Prime number – any whole number greater than 1 that has only two factors, itself and 1; that is, a number that can be divided evenly only by 1 and itself.

Composite number – any whole number greater than 1 that has more than two different factors; in other words, any whole number that is not a prime number. For example: The composite number 8 has the factors of 1, 2, 4, and 8.

Even number – any integer that can be divided by 2 without leaving a remainder. For example: 2, 4, 6, 8, and so on.

Odd number – any integer that cannot be divided evenly by 2. For example: 3, 5, 7, 9, and so on.

When you must generate questions about what the data that you have collected, you realize whether you understand it and whether you can answer your own questions. You can learn to ask yourself questions which require that you **synthesize** content from different portions of the data, such as asking questions about the data's important information.

Understanding how to **summarize** what you have collected allows you to discern what is important in the data, and to be able to express the important content in your own words. When you learn to summarize your data, you are better able to identify the main ideas of the research, and to connect these main ideas. Then, you will be better able to generate central ideas from your research. Also, you will be able to avoid irrelevant information and to remember what you have researched.

Rational numbers include all integers, decimals, and fractions. Any terminating or repeating decimal number is a rational number.

Irrational numbers cannot be written as fractions or decimals because the number of decimal places is infinite and there is no recurring pattern of digits within the number. For example, pi (π) begins with 3.141592 and continues without terminating or repeating, so pi is an irrational number.

Real numbers are the set of all rational and irrational numbers.

Decimal number – any number that uses a decimal point to show the part of the number that is less than one. Example: 1.234.

Decimal point – a symbol used to separate the ones place from the tenths place in decimals or dollars from cents in currency.

Decimal place – the position of a number to the right of the decimal point. In the decimal 0.123, the 1 is in the first place to the right of the decimal point, indicating tenths; the 2 is in the second place, indicating hundredths; and the 3 is in the third place, indicating thousandths.

The **decimal**, or base 10, system is a number system that uses ten different digits (0, 1, 2, 3, 4, 5, 6, 7, 8, 9). An example of a number system that uses something other than ten digits is the **binary**, or base 2, number system, used by computers, which uses only the numbers 0 and 1. It is thought that the decimal system originated because people had only their 10 fingers for counting.

Mathematics – Numbers and Operations

Write the place value of each digit in the following number: 14,059.826

Mathematics – Numbers and Operations

Write each number in words:
29
478
9,435
98,542
302876

Mathematics – Numbers and Operations

Write each decimal in words:
0.06
0.6
6.0
0.009
0.113
0.901

Mathematics – Numbers and Operations

Describe the parts of a fraction.

Visit *mometrix.com/academy* for a related video.
Enter video code: 262335

Mathematics – Numbers and Operations

Describe proper and improper fractions.

Mathematics – Numbers and Operations

Use a model to represent the decimal: 0.24. Write 0.24 as a fraction.

29: twenty-nine
478: four hundred seventy-eight
9,435: nine thousand four hundred thirty-five
98,542: ninety-eight thousand five hundred forty-two
302876: three hundred two thousand eight hundred seventy-six

1: ten thousands
4: thousands
0: hundreds
5: tens
9: ones
8: tenths
2: hundredths
6: thousandths

A **fraction** is a number that is expressed as one integer written above another integer, with a dividing line between them $\left(\frac{x}{y}\right)$. It represents the **quotient** of the two numbers: x divided by y. It can also be thought of as x out of y equal parts.

The top number of a fraction is called the **numerator**, and it represents the number of parts under consideration. The 1 in $\frac{1}{4}$ means that 1 part out of the whole is being considered in the calculation. The bottom number of a fraction is called the **denominator**, and it represents the total number of equal parts. The 4 in $\frac{1}{4}$ means that the whole consists of 4 equal parts. A fraction cannot have a denominator of zero; this is referred to as *undefined*.

Fractions can be manipulated, without changing the value of the fraction, by multiplying or dividing (but not adding or subtracting) both the numerator and denominator by the same number. If you divide both numbers by a common factor, you are **reducing** or simplifying the fraction. Two fractions that have the same value, but are expressed differently are known as **equivalent fractions**. For example, $\frac{2}{10}, \frac{3}{15}, \frac{4}{20}$, and $\frac{5}{25}$ are all equivalent fractions. They can also all be reduced or simplified to $\frac{1}{5}$.

0.06: six hundredths
0.6: six tenths
6.0: six
0.009: nine thousandths
0.113: one hundred thirteen thousandths
0.901: nine hundred one thousandths

The decimal 0.24 is twenty-four hundredths. One possible model to represent this fraction is to draw 100 pennies, since each penny is worth one hundredth of a dollar. Draw one hundred circles to represent one hundred pennies. Shade 24 of the pennies to represent the decimal twenty-four hundredths.

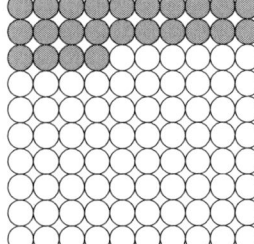

To write the decimal as a fraction, write a fraction: $\frac{\#\ shaded\ spaces}{\#\ total\ spaces}$. The number of shaded spaces is 24, and the total number of spaces is 100, so as a fraction 0.24 equals $\frac{24}{100}$. This fraction can then be reduced to $\frac{6}{25}$.

A fraction whose denominator is greater than its numerator is known as a **proper fraction**, while a fraction whose numerator is greater than its denominator is known as an **improper fraction**. Proper fractions have values *less than one* and improper fractions have values *greater than one*.

A **mixed number** is a number that contains both an integer and a fraction. Any improper fraction can be rewritten as a mixed number. Example: $\frac{8}{3} = \frac{6}{3} + \frac{2}{3} = 2 + \frac{2}{3} = 2\frac{2}{3}$. Similarly, any mixed number can be rewritten as an improper fraction. Example: $1\frac{3}{5} = 1 + \frac{3}{5} = \frac{5}{5} + \frac{3}{5} = \frac{8}{5}$.

Describe the use of percentages.

Visit *mometrix.com/academy* for a related video.
Enter video code: 693099

Describe the process of converting decimals and percentages.

Visit *mometrix.com/academy* for related videos.
Enter video codes: 306233, 986765, 696924 and 287297

Write 15% as a fraction and as a decimal.

Write 24.36% as a fraction and as a decimal.

Visit *mometrix.com/academy* for a related video.
Enter video code: 287297

Write $\frac{4}{5}$ as a decimal and as a percentage.

Write $3\frac{2}{5}$ as a decimal and as a percentage.

Visit *mometrix.com/academy* for a related video.
Enter video code: 306233

Converting decimals to percentages and percentages to decimals is as simple as moving the decimal point. To *convert from a decimal to a percentage*, move the decimal point **two places to the right**. To *convert from a percentage to a decimal*, move it **two places to the left**. Example: 0.23 = 23%; 5.34 = 534%; 0.007 = 0.7%; 700% = 7.00; 86% = 0.86; 0.15% = 0.0015.

It may be helpful to remember that the percentage number will always be larger than the equivalent decimal number.

Percentages can be thought of as fractions that are based on a whole of 100; that is, one whole is equal to 100%. The word **percent** means *per hundred*. Fractions can be expressed as percentages by finding equivalent fractions with a denomination of 100. Example: $\frac{7}{10} = \frac{70}{100} = 70\%$; $\frac{1}{4} = \frac{25}{100} = 25\%$.

To express a percentage as a fraction, divide the percentage number by 100 and reduce the fraction to its simplest possible terms. Example: $60\% = \frac{60}{100} = \frac{3}{5}$; $96\% = \frac{96}{100} = \frac{24}{25}$.

24.36% written as a fraction is $\frac{24.36}{100}$, or $\frac{2436}{10,000}$, which reduces to $\frac{609}{2500}$. 24.36% written as a decimal is 0.2436.

To convert a percentage to a fraction, follow these steps:
1. Write the percentage over 100. 15% can be written as $\frac{15}{100}$.
2. Fractions should be written in simplest form, which means that the numbers in the numerator and denominator should be reduced if possible. Both 15 and 100 can be divided by 5.
3. Therefore, $\frac{15 \div 5}{100 \div 5} = \frac{3}{20}$.

To convert a percentage to a decimal, simply remove the percent sign and move the decimal point two places to the left: 15% → 15. → 0.15

The mixed number $3\frac{2}{5}$ has a whole number and a fractional part. The fractional part $\frac{2}{5}$ can be written as a decimal by dividing 5 into 2, which gives 0.4. Adding the whole to the part gives 3.4. Alternatively, note that $3\frac{2}{5} = 3\frac{4}{10} = 3.4$.

To change a decimal to a percentage, multiply it by 100%, or equivalently move the decimal point two places to the right and add a percent sign:
$$3.4 \times 100\% = 340\%$$

Notice that this percentage is greater than 100%. This makes sense because the original mixed number $3\frac{2}{5}$ is greater than 1.

One way to convert a fraction to a decimal is to divide the numerator by the denominator:
$$\frac{4}{5} = 4 \div 5 = 0.80 = 0.8$$

Alternatively, the fraction can be manipulated to make the denominator a multiple of ten. Once the denominator is a multiple of ten, write the numerator as a decimal with as many decimal places as there are zeros in the denominator:
$$\frac{4}{5} = \frac{4 \times 2}{5 \times 2} = \frac{8}{10} = 0.8$$

Converting a decimal to a percentage may be done in much the same way as the method shown above, except that the denominator must be changed specifically to 100:
$$\frac{4 \times 20}{5 \times 20} = \frac{80}{100} = 80\%$$

Describe the 4 basic mathematical operations.

Describe the Order of Operations.

Visit *mometrix.com/academy* for a related video.
Enter video code: 259675

Evaluate the expression $5 + 20 \div 4 \times (2 + 3) - 6$ using the correct order of operations.

Describe the use of parentheses in the Order of Operations.

Describe the use of exponents.

Describe absolute values.

The **order of operations** is a set of rules that dictates the order in which we must perform each operation in an expression so that we will evaluate it accurately. If we have an expression that includes multiple different operations, the order of operations tells us which operations to do first. The most common mnemonic for the order of operations is **PEMDAS**, or "Please Excuse My Dear Aunt Sally." PEMDAS stands for parentheses, exponents, multiplication, division, addition, and subtraction. It is important to understand that multiplication and division have equal precedence, as do addition and subtraction, so those pairs of operations are simply worked from left to right in order. Example: Evaluate the expression $5 + 20 \div 4 \times (2 + 3)^2 - 6$ using the correct order of operations.

- **P:** Perform the operations inside the parentheses: $(2 + 3) = 5$
- **E:** Simplify the exponents: $(5)^2 = 5 \times 5 = 25$
    - The expression now looks like this: $5 + 20 \div 4 \times 25 - 6$
- **MD:** Perform multiplication and division from left to right: $20 \div 4 = 5$; then $5 \times 25 = 125$
    - The expression now looks like this: $5 + 125 - 6$
- **AS:** Perform addition and subtraction from left to right: $5 + 125 = 130$; then $130 - 6 = 124$

There are four basic mathematical operations:

Addition increases the value of one quantity by the value of another quantity. Example: $2 + 4 = 6; 8 + 9 = 17$. The result is called the **sum**. With addition, the order does not matter. $4 + 2 = 2 + 4$.

Subtraction is the opposite operation to addition; it decreases the value of one quantity by the value of another quantity. Example: $6 - 4 = 2; 17 - 8 = 9$. The result is called the **difference**. Note that with subtraction, the order does matter. $6 - 4 \neq 4 - 6$.

Multiplication can be thought of as repeated addition. One number tells how many times to add the other number to itself. Example: 3×2 (three times two) $= 2 + 2 + 2 = 6$. With multiplication, the order does not matter. $2 \times 3 = 3 \times 2$ or $3 + 3 = 2 + 2 + 2$.

Division is the opposite operation to multiplication; one number tells us how many parts to divide the other number into. Example: $20 \div 4 = 5$; if 20 is split into 4 equal parts, each part is 5. With division, the order of the numbers does matter. $20 \div 4 \neq 4 \div 20$.

Parentheses are used to designate which operations should be done first when there are multiple operations. Example: $4 - (2 + 1) = 1$; the parentheses tell us that we must add 2 and 1, and then subtract the sum from 4, rather than subtracting 2 from 4 and then adding 1 (this would give us an answer of 3).

- P: Perform the operations inside the parentheses: $(2 + 3) = 5$
- E: Simplify the exponents. (Not required on the ATI TEAS).
    - The equation now looks like this: $5 + 20 \div 4 \times 5 - 6$
- MD: Perform multiplication and division from left to right: $20 \div 4 = 5$; then $5 \times 5 = 25$
    - The equation now looks like this: $5 + 25 - 6$
- AS: Perform addition and subtraction from left to right: $5 + 25 = 30$; then $30 - 6 = 24$

A precursor to working with negative numbers is understanding what **absolute values** are. A number's absolute value is simply the distance away from zero a number is on the number line. The absolute value of a number is always positive and is written $|x|$.

An exponent is a superscript number placed next to another number at the top right. It indicates how many times the base number is to be multiplied by itself. **Exponents** provide a shorthand way to write what would be a longer mathematical expression. Example: $a^2 = a \times a$; $2^4 = 2 \times 2 \times 2 \times 2$. A number with an exponent of 2 is said to be **squared**, while a number with an exponent of 3 is said to be **cubed**. The value of a number raised to an exponent is called its power. So, 8^4 is read as "8 to the 4th power," or "8 raised to the power of 4." A negative exponent is the same as the **reciprocal** of a positive exponent. Example: $a^{-2} = \frac{1}{a^2}$.

Mathematics – Numbers and Operations
© Mometrix Media - flashcardsecrets.com/teas
ATI TEAS Exam

Use a number line to show that $|3| = |-3|$.

Mathematics – Numbers and Operations
© Mometrix Media - flashcardsecrets.com/teas
ATI TEAS Exam

Describe the process of addition and subtraction.

Mathematics – Numbers and Operations
© Mometrix Media - flashcardsecrets.com/teas
ATI TEAS Exam

Describe the process of multiplication and division.

Mathematics – Numbers and Operations
© Mometrix Media - flashcardsecrets.com/teas
ATI TEAS Exam

Describe the process of adding and subtracting decimals.

Visit *mometrix.com/academy* for a related video.
Enter video code: 381101

Mathematics – Numbers and Operations
© Mometrix Media - flashcardsecrets.com/teas
ATI TEAS Exam

Describe the process of multiplying decimals.

Visit *mometrix.com/academy* for a related video.
Enter video code: 731574

Mathematics – Numbers and Operations
© Mometrix Media - flashcardsecrets.com/teas
ATI TEAS Exam

Describe the process of dividing decimals.

Visit *mometrix.com/academy* for a related video.
Enter video code: 560690

Addition:
When adding signed numbers, if the signs are the same simply add the absolute values of the addends and apply the original sign to the sum. For example, $(+4) + (+8) = +12$ and $(-4) + (-8) = -12$. When the original signs are different, take the absolute values of the addends and subtract the smaller value from the larger value, then apply the original sign of the larger value to the difference. For instance, $(+4) + (-8) = -4$ and $(-4) + (+8) = +4$.

Subtraction:
For subtracting signed numbers, change the sign of the number after the minus symbol and then follow the same rules used for addition. For example, $(+4) - (+8) = (+4) + (-8) = -4$.

The absolute value of 3, written as $|3|$, is 3 because the distance between 0 and 3 on a number line is three units. Likewise, the absolute value of -3, written as $|-3|$, is 3 because the distance between 0 and -3 on a number line is three units. So, $|3| = |-3|$.

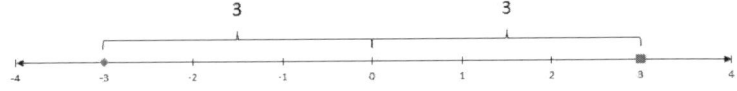

When adding and subtracting decimals, the decimal points must always be aligned. Adding decimals is just like adding regular whole numbers. Example: $4.5 + 2 = 6.5$.

If the problem-solver does not properly align the decimal points, an incorrect answer of 4.7 may result. An easy way to add decimals is to align all of the decimal points in a vertical column visually. This will allow you to see exactly where the decimal should be placed in the final answer. Begin adding from right to left. Add each column in turn, making sure to carry the number to the left if a column adds up to more than 9. The same rules apply to the subtraction of decimals.

Multiplication
If the signs are the same the product is positive when multiplying signed numbers. For example, $(+4) \times (+8) = +32$ and $(-4) \times (-8) = +32$. If the signs are opposite, the product is negative. For example, $(+4) \times (-8) = -32$ and $(-4) \times (+8) = -32$. When more than two factors are multiplied together, the sign of the product is determined by how many negative factors are present. If there are an odd number of negative factors then the product is negative, whereas an even number of negative factors indicates a positive product. For instance, $(+4) \times (-8) \times (-2) = +64$ and $(-4) \times (-8) \times (-2) = -64$.

Division
The rules for dividing signed numbers are similar to multiplying signed numbers. If the dividend and divisor have the same sign, the quotient is positive. If the dividend and divisor have opposite signs, the quotient is negative. For example, $(-4) \div (+8) = -0.5$.

Every division problem has a **divisor** and a **dividend**. The dividend is the number that is being divided. In the problem $14 \div 7$, 14 is the dividend and 7 is the divisor. In a division problem with decimals, the divisor must be converted into a whole number. Begin by moving the decimal in the divisor to the right until a whole number is created. Next, move the decimal in the dividend the same number of spaces to the right. For example, 4.9 into 24.5 would become 49 into 245. The decimal was moved one space to the right to create a whole number in the divisor, and then the same was done for the dividend. Once the whole numbers are created, the problem is carried out normally: $245 \div 49 = 5$.

A simple multiplication problem has two components: a **multiplicand** and a **multiplier**. When multiplying decimals, work as though the numbers were whole rather than decimals. Once the final product is calculated, count the number of places to the right of the decimal in both the multiplicand and the multiplier. Then, count that number of places from the right of the product and place the decimal in that position.

For example, 12.3×2.56 has three places to the right of the respective decimals. Multiply 123×256 to get 31488. Now, beginning on the right, count three places to the left and insert the decimal. The final product will be 31.488.

Mathematics – Numbers and Operations
© Mometrix Media - flashcardsecrets.com/teas
ATI TEAS Exam

Describe the process of adding and subtracting fractions.

Mathematics – Numbers and Operations
© Mometrix Media - flashcardsecrets.com/teas
ATI TEAS Exam

Describe the use of a number line.

Mathematics – Numbers and Operations
© Mometrix Media - flashcardsecrets.com/teas
ATI TEAS Exam

Name each point on the number line below:

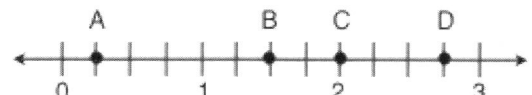

Mathematics – Numbers and Operations
© Mometrix Media - flashcardsecrets.com/teas
ATI TEAS Exam

Order the following rational numbers from least to greatest: $0.55, 17\%, \sqrt{25}, \frac{64}{4}, \frac{25}{50}, 3$.

Mathematics – Numbers and Operations
© Mometrix Media - flashcardsecrets.com/teas
ATI TEAS Exam

Order the following rational numbers from greatest to least: $0.3, 27\%, \sqrt{100}, \frac{72}{9}, \frac{1}{9}, 4.5$.

Mathematics – Numbers and Operations
© Mometrix Media - flashcardsecrets.com/teas
ATI TEAS Exam

Describe the least common denominator.

A number line is a graph to see the distance between numbers. Basically, this graph shows the relationship between numbers. So, a number line may have a point for zero and may show negative numbers on the left side of the line. Also, any positive numbers are placed on the right side of the line.

Adding and Subtracting Fractions
If two fractions have a common denominator, they can be added or subtracted simply by adding or subtracting the two numerators and retaining the same denominator. Example: $\frac{1}{2} + \frac{1}{4} = \frac{2}{4} + \frac{1}{4} = \frac{3}{4}$. If the two fractions do not already have the same denominator, one or both of them must be manipulated to achieve a common denominator before they can be added or subtracted.

Multiplying Fractions
Two fractions can be multiplied by multiplying the two numerators to find the new numerator and the two denominators to find the new denominator. Example: $\frac{1}{3} \times \frac{2}{3} = \frac{1 \times 2}{3 \times 3} = \frac{2}{9}$.

Dividing Fractions
Two fractions can be divided by flipping the numerator and denominator of the second fraction and then proceeding as though it were a multiplication. Example: $\frac{2}{3} \div \frac{3}{4} = \frac{2}{3} \times \frac{4}{3} = \frac{8}{9}$.

Recall that the term **rational** simply means that the number can be expressed as a ratio or fraction. The set of rational numbers includes integers and decimals. Notice that each of the numbers in the problem can be written as a decimal or integer:

$$17\% = 0.17$$

$$\sqrt{25} = 5$$

$$\frac{64}{4} = 16$$

$$\frac{25}{50} = \frac{1}{2} = 0.5$$

So, the answer is $17\%, \frac{25}{50}, 0.55, 3, \sqrt{25}, \frac{64}{4}$.

Use the dashed lines on the number line to identify each point. Each dashed line between two whole numbers is $\frac{1}{4}$. The line halfway between two numbers is $\frac{1}{2}$.

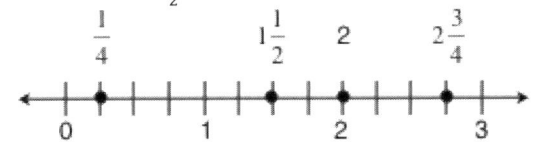

When two fractions are manipulated so that they have the same denominator, this is known as finding a **common denominator**. The number chosen to be that common denominator should be the **least common multiple** of the two original denominators. Example: $\frac{3}{4}$ and $\frac{5}{6}$; the least common multiple of 4 and 6 is 12. Manipulating to achieve the common denominator: $\frac{3}{4} = \frac{9}{12}$; $\frac{5}{6} = \frac{10}{12}$.

Recall that the term **rational** simply means that the number can be expressed as a ratio or fraction. The set of rational numbers includes integers and decimals. Notice that each of the numbers in the problem can be written as a decimal or integer:

$$27\% = 0.27$$

$$\sqrt{100} = 10$$

$$\frac{72}{9} = 8$$

$$\frac{1}{9} \approx 0.11$$

So, the answer is $\sqrt{100}, \frac{72}{9}, 4.5, 0.3, 27\%, \frac{1}{9}$.

Describe the use of factors.

Visit *mometrix.com/academy* for a related video.
Enter video code: 920086

Describe the least common multiple.

Visit *mometrix.com/academy* for a related video.
Enter video code: 838699

Describe the process of finding missing variables.

Describe what a one-variable linear equation is.

Solve for x in the following equation:

$$\frac{45\%}{12\%} = \frac{15\%}{x}$$

Solve for x in the following equation:

$$\frac{0.50}{2} = \frac{1.50}{x}$$

The least common multiple (**LCM**) is the smallest number that is a multiple of two or more numbers. For example, the multiples of 3 include 3, 6, 9, 12, 15, etc.; the multiples of 5 include 5, 10, 15, 20, etc. Therefore, the least common multiple of 3 and 5 is 15.

Factors are numbers that are multiplied together to obtain a **product**. For example, in the equation $2 \times 3 = 6$, the numbers 2 and 3 are factors. A **prime number** has only two factors (1 and itself), but other numbers can have many factors.

A **common factor** is a number that divides exactly into two or more other numbers. For example, the factors of 12 are 1, 2, 3, 4, 6, and 12, while the factors of 15 are 1, 3, 5, and 15. The common factors of 12 and 15 are 1 and 3.

A **prime factor** is also a prime number. Therefore, the prime factors of 12 are 2 and 3. For 15, the prime factors are 3 and 5.

The **greatest common factor** (**GCF**) is the largest number that is a factor of two or more numbers. For example, the factors of 15 are 1, 3, 5, and 15; the factors of 35 are 1, 5, 7, and 35. Therefore, the greatest common factor of 15 and 35 is 5.

Another way to write an equation is $ax + b = 0$ where $a \neq 0$. This is known as a **one-variable linear equation**. A solution to an equation is called a **root**.

Example: $5x + 10 = 0$

If we solve for x, the solution is $x = -2$. In other words, the root of the equation is -2.

The first step is to subtract 10 from both sides. This gives $5x = -10$. Next, divide both sides by the **coefficient** of the variable. For this example, that is 5. So, you should have $x = -2$. You can make sure that you have the correct answer by placing -2 back into the original equation. So, the equation now looks like this: $(5)(-2) + 10 = -10 + 10 = 0$.

Sometimes you will have variables missing in equations. So, you need to find the missing variable. To do this, you need to remember one important thing: *whatever you do to one side of an equation, you need to do to the other side*. If you subtract 100 from one side of an equation, you need to subtract 100 from the other side of the equation. This will allow you to change the form of the equation to find missing values.

Example
Ray earns $10 an hour. This can be given with the expression $10x$, where x is equal to the number of hours that Ray works. This is the independent variable. The independent variable is the amount that can change. The money that Ray earns is in y hours. So, you would write the equation: $10x = y$. The variable y is the dependent variable. This depends on x and cannot be changed. Now, let's say that Ray makes $360. How many hours did he work to make $360?
$$10x = 360$$
Now, you want to know how many hours that Ray worked. So, you want to get x by itself. To do that, you can divide both sides of the equation by 10.
$$\frac{10x}{10} = \frac{360}{10}$$
So, you have: $x = 36$. Now, you know that Ray worked 36 hours to make $360.

First, cross multiply; then, solve for x:

$$0.5x = 1.5 \times 2 = 3$$

$$x = \frac{3}{0.5} = 3 \times 2 = 6$$

Alternatively, notice that $\frac{0.50 \times 3}{2 \times 3} = \frac{1.50}{6}$, so $x = 6$.

First, cross multiply; then solve for x:
$$45x = 12 \times 15 = 180$$

$$x = \frac{180}{45} = 4\%$$

Alternatively, notice that $\frac{45\% \div 3}{12\% \div 3} = \frac{15\%}{4\%}$, so $x = 4\%$.

Solve for x in the following equation:

$$\frac{40}{8} = \frac{x}{24}$$

Demonstrate how to subtract 189 from 525 using regrouping.

Demonstrate how to subtract 477 from 620 using regrouping.

A patient's age is thirteen more than half of 60. How old is the patient?

A patient was given pain medicine at a dosage of 0.22 grams. The patient's dosage was then increased to 0.80 grams. By how much was the patient's dosage increased?

At a hospital, $\frac{3}{4}$ of the 100 beds are occupied today. Yesterday, $\frac{4}{5}$ of the 100 beds were occupied. On which day were more of the hospital beds occupied and by how much more?

First, set up the subtraction problem:

$$\begin{array}{r} 525 \\ -189 \\ \hline \end{array}$$

Notice that the numbers in the ones and tens columns of 525 are smaller than the numbers in the ones and tens columns of 189. This means you will need to use regrouping to perform subtraction:

$$\begin{array}{rrr} 5 & 2 & 5 \\ -1 & 8 & 9 \\ \hline \end{array}$$

To subtract 9 from 5 in the ones column you will need to borrow from the 2 in the tens columns:

$$\begin{array}{rrr} 5 & 1 & 15 \\ -1 & 8 & 9 \\ \hline & & 6 \end{array}$$

Next, to subtract 8 from 1 in the tens column you will need to borrow from the 5 in the hundreds column:

$$\begin{array}{rrr} 4 & 11 & 15 \\ -1 & 8 & 9 \\ \hline & 3 & 6 \end{array}$$

Last, subtract the 1 from the 4 in the hundreds column:

$$\begin{array}{rrr} 4 & 11 & 15 \\ -1 & 8 & 9 \\ \hline 3 & 3 & 6 \end{array}$$

First, cross multiply; then, solve for x:
$$8x = 40 \times 24 = 960$$

$$x = \frac{960}{8} = 120$$

Alternatively, notice that $\frac{40 \times 3}{8 \times 3} = \frac{120}{24}$, so $x = 120$.

The words *more than* indicate addition, and *of* indicates multiplication. The expression can be written as $\frac{1}{2} \times 60 + 13$, so the patient's age is $\frac{1}{2} \times 60 + 13 = 30 + 13 = 43$. The patient is 43 years old.

First, set up the subtraction problem:

$$\begin{array}{r} 620 \\ -477 \\ \hline \end{array}$$

Notice that the numbers in the ones and tens columns of 620 are smaller than the numbers in the ones and tens columns of 477. This means you will need to use regrouping to perform subtraction:

$$\begin{array}{rrr} 6 & 2 & 0 \\ -4 & 7 & 7 \\ \hline \end{array}$$

To subtract 7 from 0 in the ones column you will need to borrow from the 2 in the tens column:

$$\begin{array}{rrr} 6 & 1 & 10 \\ -4 & 7 & 7 \\ \hline & & 3 \end{array}$$

Next, to subtract 7 from the 1 that's still in the tens column you will need to borrow from the 6 in the hundreds column:

$$\begin{array}{rrr} 5 & 11 & 10 \\ -4 & 7 & 7 \\ \hline & 4 & 3 \end{array}$$

Lastly, subtract 4 from the 5 remaining in the hundreds column:

$$\begin{array}{rrr} 5 & 11 & 10 \\ -4 & 7 & 7 \\ \hline 1 & 4 & 3 \end{array}$$

First, find the number of beds that were occupied each day. To do so, multiply the fraction of beds occupied by the number of beds available:

Number of beds occupied today $= \frac{3}{4} \times 100 = 75$.

Number of beds occupied yesterday $= \frac{4}{5} \times 100 = 80$.

The difference in the number of beds occupied is $80 - 75 = 5$ beds.

Therefore, 5 more beds were occupied yesterday than today.

The first step is to determine what operation (addition, subtraction, multiplication, or division) the problem requires. Notice the key words and phrases *by how much* and *increased*. This indicates that you are looking for the amount of change or the difference between the two amounts. This difference is found by subtracting the smaller amount from the larger amount. Remember to line up the decimal when subtracting:

$$\begin{array}{r} 0.80 \\ -0.22 \\ \hline 0.58 \end{array}$$

At a hospital, 40% of the nurses work in labor and delivery. If 20 nurses work in labor and delivery, how many nurses work at the hospital?

A patient was given blood pressure medicine at a dosage of 2 grams. The patient's dosage was then decreased to 0.45 grams. By how much was the patient's dosage decreased?

Two weeks ago, $\frac{2}{3}$ of the 60 patients at a hospital were male. Last week, $\frac{3}{6}$ of the 80 patients were male. During which week were there more male patients?

Jane ate lunch at a local restaurant. She ordered a $4.99 appetizer, a $12.50 entrée, and a $1.25 soda. If she wants to tip her server 20%, how much money will she spend in all?

Explain the components of percentage problems.

Visit *mometrix.com/academy* for a related video.
Enter video code: 538674

What is 30% of 120?

The decrease is represented by the difference between the two amounts. Remember to line up the decimal point before subtracting:

$$\begin{array}{r} 2.00 \\ -0.45 \\ \hline 1.55 \end{array}$$

To answer this problem, first think about the number of nurses that work at the hospital. Will it be more or less than the number of nurses who work in a specific department such as labor and delivery? More nurses work at the hospital, so the number you find to answer this question will be greater than 20.

40% of the nurses are labor and delivery nurses. The word *of* indicates multiplication, and the words *is* and *are* indicate equivalence. Translating the problem into a mathematical sentence gives $40\% \times n = 20$, where n represents the total number of nurses. Solving for n gives $n = \frac{20}{40\%} = \frac{20}{0.40} = 50$. Fifty nurses work at the hospital.

To find total amount, first find the sum of the items she ordered from the menu and then add 20% of this sum to the total:

$$\$4.99 + \$12.50 + \$1.25 = \$18.74$$

$$\$18.74 \times 20\% = \$18.74 \times 0.2 = \$3.748 \approx \$3.75$$

$$\text{Total} = \$18.74 + \$3.75 = \$22.49$$

Another way to find this sum is to multiply the cost of the meal by 120%:

$$\$18.74 \times 120\% = \$18.74 \times 1.2 = \$22.488 \approx \$22.49$$

First, you need to find the number of male patients that were in the hospital each week. You are given this amount in terms of fractions. To find the number of male patients, multiply the fraction of male patients by the number of patients in the hospital.

Number of male patients = fraction of male patients × total number of patients.

Number of male patients two weeks ago $= \frac{2}{3} \times 60 = \frac{120}{3} = 40$.

Number of male patients last week $= \frac{3}{6} \times 80 = \frac{1}{2} \times 80 = \frac{80}{2} = 40$.

The number of male patients was the same both weeks.

The word *of* indicates multiplication, so 30% of 120 is found by multiplying 120 by 30%. Change 30% to a fraction or decimal, then multiply:

$$30\% = \frac{30}{100} = 0.3$$

$$120 \times 0.3 = 36$$

A percentage problem can be presented three main ways: (1) Find what percentage of some number another number is. Example: What percentage of 40 is 8? (2) Find what number is some percentage of a given number. Example: What number is 20% of 40? (3) Find what number another number is a given percentage of. Example: What number is 8 20% of?

The three components in all of these cases are the same: a **whole** (W), a **part** (P), and a **percentage** (%). These are related by the equation: $P = W \times \%$. This is the form of the equation you would use to solve problems of type (2). To solve types (1) and (3), you would use these two forms: $\% = \frac{P}{W}$ and $W = \frac{P}{\%}$

The thing that frequently makes percentage problems difficult is that they are most often also word problems, so a large part of solving them is figuring out which quantities are what. Example: In a school cafeteria, 7 students choose pizza, 9 choose hamburgers, and 4 choose tacos. Find the percentage that chooses tacos. To find the whole, you must first add all of the parts: $7 + 9 + 4 = 20$. The percentage can then be found by dividing the part by the whole $\left(\% = \frac{P}{W}\right)$: $\frac{4}{20} = \frac{20}{100} = 20\%$.

Mathematics – Numbers and Operations
© Mometrix Media - flashcardsecrets.com/teas
ATI TEAS Exam

What is 150% of 20?

Mathematics – Numbers and Operations
© Mometrix Media - flashcardsecrets.com/teas
ATI TEAS Exam

What is 14.5% of 96?

Mathematics – Numbers and Operations
© Mometrix Media - flashcardsecrets.com/teas
ATI TEAS Exam

According to a hospital survey, 82% of nurses were highly satisfied at their job. Of 145 nurses, how many were highly satisfied?

Mathematics – Numbers and Operations
© Mometrix Media - flashcardsecrets.com/teas
ATI TEAS Exam

During a shift, a new nurse spent five hours of her time observing procedures, three hours working in the oncology department, and four hours doing paperwork. During the next shift, she spent four hours observing procedures, six hours in the oncology department, and two hours doing paperwork. What was the percent change for each task between the two shifts?

Mathematics – Numbers and Operations
© Mometrix Media - flashcardsecrets.com/teas
ATI TEAS Exam

A patient was given 40 mg of a certain medicine. Later, the patient's dosage was increased to 45 mg. What was the percent increase in his medication?

Mathematics – Numbers and Operations
© Mometrix Media - flashcardsecrets.com/teas
ATI TEAS Exam

A patient was given 100 mg of a certain medicine. The patient's dosage was later decreased to 88 mg. What was the percent decrease?

Change 14.5% to a decimal and multiply:

$$0.145 \times 96 = 13.92$$

Notice that 13.92 is much smaller than the original number of 96. This makes sense because you are finding a small percentage of the original number.

The word *of* indicates multiplication, so 150% of 20 is found by multiplying 20 by 150%. Change 150% to a fraction or decimal, then multiply:

$$150\% = \frac{150}{100} = 1.5$$

$$20 \times 1.5 = 30$$

Notice that 30 is greater than the original number of 20. This makes sense because you are finding a number that is more than 100% of the original number.

The three tasks are observing procedures, working in the oncology department, and doing paperwork. To find the amount of change, compare the first amount with the second amount for each task. Then, write this difference as a percentage compared to the initial amount.
Amount of change for observing procedures: 5 hr − 4 hr = 1 hr.
The percent of change is $\frac{\text{amount of change}}{\text{original amount}} \times 100\%$. $\frac{1 \text{ hour}}{5 \text{ hours}} \times 100\% = 20\%$.
The nurse spent 20% less time observing procedures on her second shift than on her first.
Amount of change for working in the oncology department: 6 hr − 3 hr = 3 hr.
The percent of change is $\frac{\text{amount of change}}{\text{original amount}} \times 100\%$. $\frac{3 \text{ hours}}{3 \text{ hours}} \times 100\% = 100\%$. The nurse spent 100% more time (or twice as much time) working in the oncology department during her second shift than she did in her first.
Amount of change for doing paperwork: 4 hr − 2 hr = 2 hr.
The percent of change is $\frac{\text{amount of change}}{\text{original amount}} \times 100\%$. $\frac{2 \text{ hours}}{4 \text{ hours}} \times 100\% = 50\%$.
The nurse spent 50% less time (or half as much time) working on paperwork during her second shift than she did in her first.

Write 82% of 145 as an equation:

$$0.82 \times 145 = 118.9$$

Because you can't have 0.9 of a person, the answer is, "About 119 nurses are highly satisfied with their jobs."

The medication was decreased by 12 mg (100 mg − 88 mg = 12 mg). To find by what percent the medication was decreased, this change must be written as a percentage when compared to the original amount.
In other words, $\frac{\text{original amount} - \text{new amount}}{\text{original amount}} \times 100\% = $ percent decrease

$$\frac{12 \text{ mg}}{100 \text{ mg}} \times 100\% = 0.12 \times 100\% = 12\%$$

The percent decrease is 12%.

To find the percent increase, first compare the original and increased amounts. The original amount was 40 mg, and the increased amount is 45 mg, so the dosage of medication was increased by 5 mg (45 − 40 = 5). Note, however, that the question asks not by how much the dosage increased but by what percentage it increased. Percent increase = $\frac{\text{new amount} - \text{original amount}}{\text{original amount}} \times 100\%$.

$$\frac{45 \text{ mg} - 40 \text{ mg}}{40 \text{ mg}} \times 100\% = \frac{5}{40} \times 100\% = 0.125 \times 100\% = 12.5\%$$

The percent increase is 12.5%.

Mathematics – Numbers and Operations

A patient complaining of fatigue and weight gain was diagnosed with hypothyroidism and was prescribed 125 mcg of medication. Three months later, her symptoms had improved, and her thyroid stimulation hormone (TSH) level was found to be 0.5 mIU/L. The doctor reduced the patient's thyroid medication dosage to 100 mcg, after which the patient's TSH level was found to be 1.5 mIU/L, which is within the normal range. By what percentage did the doctor reduce the patient's thyroid medication?

Mathematics – Numbers and Operations

In a performance review, an employee received a score of 70 for efficiency and 90 for meeting project deadlines. Six months later, the employee received a score of 65 for efficiency and 96 for meeting project deadlines. What was the percent change for each score on the performance review?

Mathematics – Numbers and Operations

Explain what rounding is.

Mathematics – Numbers and Operations

Describe the process of rounding.

Mathematics – Numbers and Operations

E Estimate the sum of 345,932 and 96,369 by rounding each number to the nearest ten thousand.

Mathematics – Numbers and Operations

A patient's heart beat 422 times over the course of six minutes. About how many times did the patient's heart beat during each minute?

To find the percent change, compare the first amount with the second amount for each score; then, write this difference as a percentage of the initial amount.

Percent change for efficiency score:
$$70 - 65 = 5; \quad \frac{5}{70} \approx 7.1\%$$
The employee's efficiency decreased by about 7.1%.

Percent change for meeting project deadlines score:
$$96 - 90 = 6; \quad \frac{6}{90} \approx 6.7\%$$
The employee increased his ability to meet project deadlines by about 6.7%.

In this problem you must determine which information is necessary to answer the question. The question asks by what percentage the doctor reduced the patient's thyroid medication dosage. Find the two dosage amounts and perform subtraction to find their difference. The first dosage amount is 125 mcg. The second dosage amount is 100 mcg. Therefore, the difference is 125 mcg − 100 mcg = 25 mcg. The percentage reduction can then be calculated as $\frac{\text{change}}{\text{original}} = \frac{25 \text{ mcg}}{125 \text{ mcg}} = \frac{1}{5} = 20\%$.

Rounding is reducing the digits in a number while still trying to keep the value similar. The result will be less accurate, but it will be in a simpler form and will be easier to use. Whole numbers can be **rounded** to the nearest ten, hundred, thousand, etc.
1. Remember, when rounding to the nearest ten, anything ending in 5 or greater rounds up. So, 11 rounds to 10, 47 rounds to 50, and 118 rounds to 120.
2. Remember, when rounding to the nearest hundred, anything ending in 50 or greater rounds up. So, 78 rounds to 100, 980 rounds to 1000, and 248 rounds to 200.
3. Remember, when rounding to the nearest thousand, anything ending in 500 or greater rounds up. So, 302 rounds to 0, 1274 rounds to 1000, and 3756 rounds to 4000.

When you are asked to estimate the solution a problem, you will need to provide only an approximate figure or **estimation** for your answer. In this situation, you will need to round each number in the calculation to the level indicated (nearest hundred, nearest thousand, etc.) or to a level that makes sense for the numbers involved. When estimating a sum **all numbers must be rounded to the same level**. You cannot round one number to the nearest thousand while rounding another to the nearest hundred.

Rounding is reducing the number of non-zero digits in a number while trying to keep the value similar to what it was before. The result will be less accurate, but it will be in a simpler form and will be easier to use. Numbers can be **rounded** to the nearest ten, hundred, thousand, etc.

The words *about how many* indicate that you need to estimate the solution. In this case, look at the numbers you are given. 422 can be rounded down to 420, which is easily divisible by 6. A good estimate is 420 ÷ 6 = 70 beats per minute. More accurately, the patient's average heart rate was just over 70 beats per minute since his heart actually beat a little more than 420 times in six minutes.

Start by rounding each number to the nearest ten thousand: 345,932 becomes 350,000, and 96,369 becomes 100,000.

Then, add the rounded numbers: 350,000 + 100,000 = 450,000. So, the answer is approximately 450,000.

The exact answer would be 345,932 + 96,369 = 442,301. So, the estimate of 450,000 is a similar value to the exact answer.

Describe what a proportion is.

Describe what a ratio is.

Visit *mometrix.com/academy* for a related video.
Enter video code: 996914

A patient receives 100 mg of a medication every two hours. How much medication does the patient receive on average in five hours?

At a hospital, for every 20 female patients there are 15 male patients. This same patient ratio happens to exist at another hospital. If there are 100 female patients at the second hospital, how many male patients are there?

In a hospital emergency room, there are 4 nurses for every 12 patients. What is the ratio of nurses to patients? If the nurse-to-patient ratio remains constant, how many nurses must be present to care for 24 patients?

In an intensive care unit, the nurse-to-patient ratio is 1:2. If seven nurses are on duty, how many patients are currently in the ICU?

A ratio is a comparison of two quantities in a particular order. Example: If there are 14 computers in a lab, and the class has 20 students, there is a student to computer **ratio** of 20 to 14, commonly written as 20:14. Ratios are normally reduced to their smallest whole number representation, so 20:14 would be reduced to 10:7 by dividing both sides by 2.

A proportion is a relationship between two quantities that dictates how one changes when the other changes. A **direct proportion** describes a relationship in which a quantity increases by a set amount for every increase in the other quantity, or decreases by that same amount for every decrease in the other quantity. Example: Assuming a constant driving speed, the time required for a car trip increases as the distance of the trip increases. The distance to be traveled and the time required to travel are directly proportional.

An **inverse proportion** is a relationship in which an increase in one quantity is accompanied by a decrease in the other, or vice versa. Example: the time required for a car trip decreases as the speed increases, and increases as the speed decreases, so the time required is inversely proportional to the speed of the car.

One way to find the number of male patients is to set up and solve a proportion.

$$\frac{\text{number of female patients}}{\text{number of male patients}} = \frac{20}{15} = \frac{100}{x}$$

Cross multiply and then solve for x:

$$20x = 15 \times 100 = 1500$$

$$x = \frac{1500}{20} = 75$$

Alternatively, notice that: $\frac{20 \times 5}{15 \times 5} = \frac{100}{75}$, so $x = 75$.

Using proportional reasoning, since five hours is 2.5 times as long as two hours, the patient will receive two and a half times as much medication: 2.5×100 mg $= 250$ mg, in five hours.

To compute the answer methodically, create two ratios for medication over time—one for the given values, and one that includes the missing value:

$$\frac{\text{medication}}{\text{time}} = \frac{100 \text{ mg}}{2 \text{ hr}} = \frac{x \text{ mg}}{5 \text{ hr}}$$

Cross multiply, and then solve for x:

$$2x = 100 \times 5 = 500$$

$$x = \frac{500}{2} = 250$$

Therefore, the patient receives 250 mg every five hours.

Use proportional reasoning or set up a proportion to solve. Because there are twice as many patients as nurses, there must be fourteen patients when seven nurses are on duty. Setting up and solving a proportion gives the same result:

$$\frac{\text{number of nurses}}{\text{number of patients}} = \frac{1}{2} = \frac{7}{x}$$

Cross multiply, then solve for x:

$$x = 7 \times 2 = 14$$

The ratio of nurses to patients can be written as 4 to 12, 4:12, or $\frac{4}{12}$. Because four and twelve have a common factor of four, the ratio should be reduced to 1:3, which means that there is one nurse present for every three patients. If this ratio remains constant, there must be eight nurses present to care for 24 patients.

Mathematics – Numbers and Operations

Describe the constant of proportionality.

Mathematics – Numbers and Operations

Describe how to find the slope of a graph with two points.

Mathematics – Numbers and Operations

Provide an example of a real-world proportional relationship.

Mathematics – Numbers and Operations

Describe the term unit rate.

Mathematics – Numbers and Operations

Janice made $40 during the first 5 hours she spent babysitting. She will continue to earn money at this rate until she finishes babysitting in 3 more hours. Find how much money Janice earned babysitting and how much she earns per hour.

Mathematics – Numbers and Operations

The McDonalds are taking a family road trip, driving 300 miles to their cabin. It took them 2 hours to drive the first 120 miles. They will drive at the same speed all the way to their cabin. Find the speed at which the McDonalds are driving and how much longer it will take them to get to their cabin.

On a graph with two points, (x_1, y_1) and (x_2, y_2), the **slope** m is found with the formula $m = \frac{y_2 - y_1}{x_2 - x_1}$; where $x_1 \neq x_2$. If the value of the slope is **positive**, the line has an *upward direction* from left to right. If the value of the slope is **negative**, the line has a *downward direction* from left to right.

When two quantities have a proportional relationship, there exists a **constant of proportionality** between the quantities. The product of this constant and one of the quantities is equal to the other quantity. For example, if one lemon costs $0.25, two lemons cost $0.50, and three lemons cost $0.75, there is a proportional relationship between the total cost of lemons and the number of lemons purchased. The constant of proportionality is the **unit price**, namely $0.25/lemon. Notice that the total price of lemons, t, can be found by multiplying the unit price of lemons, p, and the number of lemons, n: $t = pn$.

Unit rate expresses a quantity of one thing in terms of one unit of another. For example, if you travel 30 miles every two hours, a **unit rate** expresses this comparison in terms of one hour: in one hour you travel 15 miles, so your unit rate is 15 miles per hour. Other examples are how much one ounce of food costs (price per ounce), or figuring out how much one egg costs out of the dozen (price per 1 egg, instead of price per 12 eggs). The denominator of a unit rate is always 1.

Unit rates are used to compare different options to solve problems. For example, to make sure you get the best deal when deciding which kind of soda to buy, you can find the unit rate of each. If soda #1 costs $1.50 for a 1-liter bottle, and soda #2 costs $2.75 for a 2-liter bottle, it would be a better deal to buy soda #2, because its unit rate is only $1.375 per liter, which is cheaper than soda #1.

Unit rates can also help determine the length of time a given event will take. For example, if you can paint 2 rooms in 4.5 hours, you can determine how long it will take you to paint 5 rooms by solving for the unit rate per room and then multiplying by 5.

$$\text{unit rate} = \frac{4.5 \text{ hr}}{2 \text{ rooms}} = 2.25 \frac{\text{hr}}{\text{room}}$$
$$5 \times \text{unit rate} = 5 \times 2.25 = 11.25 \text{ hr}$$

A new book goes on sale. In the first month, 5,000 copies of the book are sold. Over time, the book maintains its popularity. The data for the number of copies sold is in the table below.

# of Months on Sale	1	2	3	4	5
# of Copies Sold (Thousands)	5	10	15	20	25

So, the number of copies that are sold and the time that the book is on sale have a proportional relationship. In this example, an equation can be used to show the data: $y = 5x$, where x is the number of months that the book is on sale, and y is the number of copies sold. The slope is $\frac{rise}{run} = \frac{5}{1}$, which can be reduced to 5.

The McDonalds' speed can be found by dividing the distance traveled by the time it took to travel:

$$\text{Speed} = \frac{120 \text{ mi}}{2 \text{ hr}} = 60 \text{ mph}$$

To determine the amount of time it will take for them to drive the rest of the way, first find how many miles they have left: $300 - 120 = 180$ mi. Divide the remaining distance by the rate of travel to find the remaining travel time:

$$\text{Time} = \frac{180 \text{ mi}}{60 \text{ mph}} = 3 \text{ hr}$$

The total Janice will earn can be found by setting up a proportion comparing money earned to babysitting hours. Since she earned $40 for 5 hours and since the rate is constant, she will earn a proportional amount in 8 hours: $\frac{40}{5} = \frac{x}{8}$. Cross multiplying yields $5x = 8 \times 40 = 320$, and division by 5 shows that $x = \frac{320}{5} = 64$. Janice made a total of $64. The hourly rate can be found by taking her total amount earned and dividing it by the number of hours worked. Since $\frac{64}{8} = 8$, Janice makes $8 per hour.

Mathematics – Numbers and Operations
© Mometrix Media - flashcardsecrets.com/teas
ATI TEAS Exam

It takes Andy 10 minutes to read 6 pages of his book. He has already read 150 pages in his book that is 210 pages long. Find how long it takes Andy to read 1 page and also find how long it will take him to finish his book if he continues to read at the same speed.

Mathematics – Numbers and Operations
© Mometrix Media - flashcardsecrets.com/teas
ATI TEAS Exam

Describe the process of writing out an inequality.

Mathematics – Numbers and Operations
© Mometrix Media - flashcardsecrets.com/teas
ATI TEAS Exam

A farm sells vegetables and dairy products. One third of the sales from dairy products plus half of the sales from vegetables should be greater than the monthly payment (P) for the farm.

Mathematics – Numbers and Operations
© Mometrix Media - flashcardsecrets.com/teas
ATI TEAS Exam

John and Luke play basketball every week. John shoots free throws while Luke shoots three-point shots. John can make 5 more shots per minute than Luke. On one day, John made 30 free throws in the same time that it took Luke to make 20 three-point shots. How fast are Luke and John making shots?

Mathematics – Numbers and Operations
© Mometrix Media - flashcardsecrets.com/teas
ATI TEAS Exam

Fred buys some CDs for $12 each. He also buys two DVDs. The total that Fred spent is $60. Write an equation that shows the connection between the number of CDs and the average cost of a DVD.

Mathematics – Numbers and Operations
© Mometrix Media - flashcardsecrets.com/teas
ATI TEAS Exam

Simplify the inequality $7x > 5$.

= **is**, was, were, will be, equals, is equal to, yields, is the same as, amounts to, becomes
> **is** greater than, **is** more than
≥ **is** greater than or equal to, is at least, is no less than
< **is** less than, **is** fewer than
≤ **is** less than or equal to, is at most, is no more than

To write out an **inequality**, you may need to translate a sentence into an inequality. This translation is putting the words into symbols. When translating, choose a variable to stand for the unknown value. Then, change the words or phrases into symbols. For example, the sum of 2 and a number is at most 12. So, you would write: $2 + b \leq 12$.

Andy's reading time per page can be found by dividing the time it takes him to read 6 pages by 6:

$$Rate = \frac{10}{6} = \frac{5}{3} = 1\frac{2}{3} \text{ min} = 1 \text{ min}, 40 \text{ sec per page}$$

The time it will take Andy to finish the book can be found by first figuring out how many pages he has left to read, and then multiplying this number by his reading time per page:

$$210 - 150 = 60 \text{ pages}$$

$$60 \times \frac{5}{3} = \frac{300}{3} = 100 \text{ min} = 1 \text{ hr}, 40 \text{ min}$$

First, determine what you know and what values you can set as equal to each other. You know how many shots each player made in an unknown time period and their rate relative to the other player. The values that can be set as equal are the times it took each player to make their shots. Even though you don't know the value for the time, you know it's the same for both players. When you have a quantity and a rate, dividing the quantity by the rate gives you the time. So divide each player's number of made shots by their rate and set those values equal. Luke made 20 shots at a rate of x shots per minute: $\frac{20}{x}$. John made 30 shots at a rate of $x + 5$ shots per minute (he made 5 shots per minute more than Luke): $\frac{30}{x+5}$. Set these two values equal to one another because they both represent the amount of time it took to make the shots:

$$\frac{30}{x+5} = \frac{20}{x}$$

Cross multiply the proportion: $30x = 20(x + 5)$

Distribute the 20 across the parentheses: $30x = 20x + 100$

Subtract $20x$ from both sides of the equation, and you are left with: $10x = 100$

Divide both sides by 10: $x = \frac{100}{10} = 10$

Luke's speed was 10 three-point shots per minute, so John's speed was 15 free throws per minute.

Let d stand for the sales from dairy products. Let v stand for the sales from vegetables. One third of the sales from dairy products is the expression $\frac{d}{3}$. One half of the sales from vegetables is the expression $\frac{v}{2}$. The sum of these expressions should be greater than the monthly payment for the farm. An inequality for this is $\frac{d}{3} + \frac{v}{2} > P$.

Solving inequalities can be done with the same rules as for solving equations. However, when multiplying or dividing by a negative number, the direction of the **inequality sign** must be flipped or **reversed**.

To solve for x, divide both sides by 7:

$$x > \frac{5}{7}$$

Let c stand for the number of CDs that Fred buys. Also, let D stand for the cost of each DVD that Fred buys. The expression $12c$ gives the cost of the CDs, and the expression $2D$ gives the cost of the DVDs. So the equation $12c + 2D = 60$ represents the situation described.

Mathematics – Numbers and Operations
© Mometrix Media - flashcardsecrets.com/teas
ATI TEAS Exam

Graph the inequality $10 > -2x + 4$.

Mathematics – Numbers and Operations
© Mometrix Media - flashcardsecrets.com/teas
ATI TEAS Exam

Simplify the following expression:

$$\frac{\frac{2}{5}}{\frac{4}{7}}$$

Mathematics – Numbers and Operations
© Mometrix Media - flashcardsecrets.com/teas
ATI TEAS Exam

Simplify the following expression:

$$\frac{1}{4} + \frac{3}{6}$$

Mathematics – Numbers and Operations
© Mometrix Media - flashcardsecrets.com/teas
ATI TEAS Exam

Simplify the following expression:

$$\frac{7}{8} - \frac{8}{16}$$

Mathematics – Numbers and Operations
© Mometrix Media - flashcardsecrets.com/teas
ATI TEAS Exam

Simplify the following expression:

$$\frac{1}{2} + \left(3\left(\frac{3}{4}\right) - 2\right) + 4$$

Mathematics – Numbers and Operations
© Mometrix Media - flashcardsecrets.com/teas
ATI TEAS Exam

Simplify the following expression:

$$0.22 + 0.5 - (5.5 + 3.3 \div 3)$$

Dividing a fraction by a fraction may appear tricky, but it's not if you write out your steps carefully. Follow these steps to divide a fraction by a fraction.

Step 1: Rewrite the problem as a multiplication problem. Dividing by a fraction is the same as multiplying by its **reciprocal**, also known as its **multiplicative inverse**. The product of a number and its reciprocal is 1. Because $\frac{4}{7}$ times $\frac{7}{4}$ is 1, these numbers are reciprocals. Note that reciprocals can be found by simply interchanging the numerators and denominators. So, rewriting the problem as a multiplication problem gives $\frac{2}{5} \times \frac{7}{4}$.

Step 2: Perform multiplication of the fractions by multiplying the numerators by each other and the denominators by each other. In other words, multiply across the top and then multiply across the bottom.

$$\frac{2}{5} \times \frac{7}{4} = \frac{2 \times 7}{5 \times 4} = \frac{14}{20}$$

Step 3: Make sure the fraction is reduced to lowest terms. Both 14 and 20 can be divided by 2.

$$\frac{14}{20} = \frac{14 \div 2}{20 \div 2} = \frac{7}{10}$$

The answer is $\frac{7}{10}$.

In order to graph the inequality $10 > -2x + 4$, you need to solve for x. The opposite of addition is subtraction. So, subtract 4 from both sides. This gives you $6 > -2x$. Next, the opposite of multiplication is division. So, divide both sides by -2. Don't forget to flip the inequality symbol because you are dividing by a negative number. Now, you have $-3 < x$. You can rewrite this as $x > -3$.

To graph an inequality, you make a **number line**. Then, put a circle around the value that is being compared to x. If you are graphing a *greater than* or *less than* inequality, the circle remains open. This represents all of the values up to, but not including, -3. If the inequality is *greater than or equal to* or *less than or equal to*, you draw a closed circle around the value. This would represent all of the values up to, and including, the number. Finally, look over the values that the solution stands for. Then, shade the number line in the needed direction. This example calls for graphing all of the values greater than -3. This is all of the numbers to the right of -3, so you would then shade this area on the number line.

Fractions with common denominators can be easily added or subtracted. Recall that the denominator is the bottom number in the fraction and that the numerator is the top number in the fraction.

The denominators of $\frac{7}{8}$ and $\frac{8}{16}$ are 8 and 16, respectively. The lowest common denominator of 8 and 16 is 16 because 16 is the least common multiple of 8 (multiples 8, 16, 24 ...) and 16 (multiples 16, 32, 48, ...). Convert each fraction to its equivalent with the newly found common denominator of 16.

$$\frac{7 \times 2}{8 \times 2} = \frac{14}{16} \qquad \frac{8 \times 1}{16 \times 1} = \frac{8}{16}$$

Now that the fractions have the same denominator, you can subtract them.

$$\frac{14}{16} - \frac{8}{16} = \frac{6}{16}$$

Be sure to write your answer in lowest terms. Both 6 and 16 can be divided by 2, so the answer is $\frac{3}{8}$.

Fractions with common denominators can be easily added or subtracted. Recall that the denominator is the bottom number in the fraction and that the numerator is the top number in the fraction.

The denominators of $\frac{1}{4}$ and $\frac{3}{6}$ are 4 and 6, respectively. The lowest common denominator of 4 and 6 is 12 because 12 is the least common multiple of 4 (multiples 4, 8, 12, 16, ...) and 6 (multiples 6, 12, 18, 24, ...). Convert each fraction to its equivalent with the newly found common denominator of 12.

$$\frac{1 \times 3}{4 \times 3} = \frac{3}{12}; \frac{3 \times 2}{6 \times 2} = \frac{6}{12}.$$

Now that the fractions have the same denominator, you can add them.

$$\frac{3}{12} + \frac{6}{12} = \frac{9}{12}.$$

Be sure to write your answer in lowest terms. Both 9 and 12 can be divided by 3, so the answer is $\frac{3}{4}$.

First, evaluate the terms in the parentheses $(5.5 + 3.3 \div 3)$ using order of operations. $3.3 \div 3 = 1.1$, and $5.5 + 1.1 = 6.6$.

Next, rewrite the problem: $0.22 + 0.5 - 6.6$.

Finally, add and subtract from left to right: $0.22 + 0.5 = 0.72$; $0.72 - 6.6 = -5.88$. The answer is -5.88.

When simplifying expressions, first perform operations within groups. Within the set of parentheses are multiplication and subtraction operations. Perform the multiplication first to get $\frac{1}{2} + \left(\frac{9}{4} - 2\right) + 4$. Then, subtract two to obtain $\frac{1}{2} + \frac{1}{4} + 4$. Finally, perform addition from left to right: $\frac{1}{2} + \frac{1}{4} + 4 = \frac{2}{4} + \frac{1}{4} + \frac{16}{4} = \frac{19}{4}$.

Mathematics – Numbers and Operations
© Mometrix Media - flashcardsecrets.com/teas
ATI TEAS Exam

Simplify the following expression:

$$\frac{3}{2} + (4(0.5) - 0.75) + 2$$

Mathematics – Numbers and Operations
© Mometrix Media - flashcardsecrets.com/teas
ATI TEAS Exam

Simplify the following expression:

$$1.45 + 1.5 + (6 - 9 \div 2) + 45$$

Mathematics – Data Interpretation
© Mometrix Media - flashcardsecrets.com/teas
ATI TEAS Exam

Describe the use of statistics.

Mathematics – Data Interpretation
© Mometrix Media - flashcardsecrets.com/teas
ATI TEAS Exam

Describe the use of a bar graph.

Mathematics – Data Interpretation
© Mometrix Media - flashcardsecrets.com/teas
ATI TEAS Exam

Describe the use of a line graph.

Mathematics – Data Interpretation
© Mometrix Media - flashcardsecrets.com/teas
ATI TEAS Exam

Describe the use of a pictograph.

First, evaluate the terms in the parentheses using proper order of operations.

$$1.45 + 1.5 + (6 - 4.5) + 45$$
$$1.45 + 1.5 + 1.5 + 45$$

Finally, add from left to right.

$$1.45 + 1.5 + 1.5 + 45 = 49.45$$

First change the fraction to a decimal:

$$1.5 + (4(0.5) - 0.75) + 2$$
$$1.5 + (2 - 0.75) + 2$$

Then perform addition from left to right:

$$1.5 + 1.25 + 2 = 4.75$$

A **bar graph** is a graph that uses bars to compare data, as if each bar were a ruler being used to measure the data. The graph includes a **scale** that identifies the units being measured.

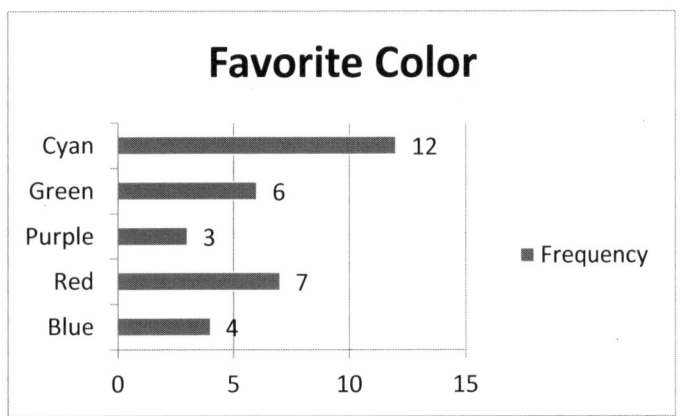

Statistics is the branch of mathematics that deals with collecting, recording, interpreting, illustrating, and analyzing large amounts of **data**. The following terms are often used in the discussion of data and **statistics**:

- **Data** – the collective name for pieces of *information* (singular is datum).
- **Quantitative data** – measurements (such as length, mass, and speed) that provide information about *quantities* in numbers
- **Qualitative data** – information (such as colors, scents, tastes, and shapes) that *cannot be measured* using numbers
- **Discrete data** – information that can be expressed only by a *specific value*, such as whole or half numbers. For example, since people can be counted only in whole numbers, a population count would be discrete data.
- **Continuous data** – information (such as time and temperature) that can be expressed by *any value within a given range*
- **Primary data** – information that has been *collected* directly from a survey, investigation, or experiment, such as a questionnaire or the recording of daily temperatures. Primary data that has not yet been organized or analyzed is called raw data.
- **Secondary data** – information that has been collected, sorted, and *processed* by the researcher
- **Ordinal data** – information that *can be placed in numerical order*, such as age or weight
- **Nominal data** – information that *cannot be placed in numerical order*, such as names or places.

A **pictograph** is a graph that uses pictures or symbols to show data. The pictograph will have a key to identify what each symbol represents. Generally, each symbol stands for one or more objects.

A **line graph** is a graph that connects points to show how data increases or decreases over time. The time line is the **horizontal axis**. The connecting lines between data points on the graph are a way to more clearly show how the data changes.

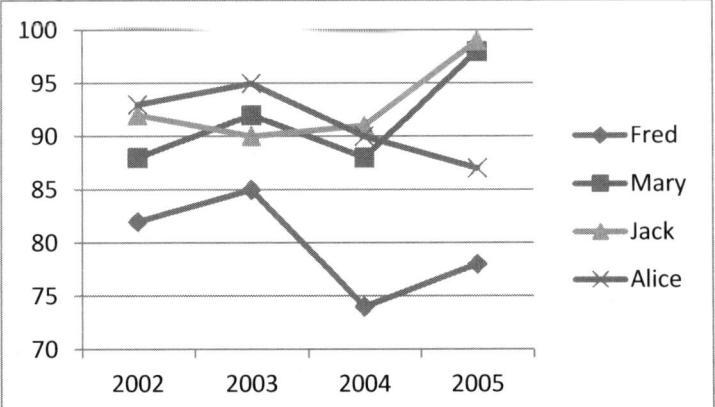

Mathematics – Data Interpretation
© Mometrix Media - flashcardsecrets.com/teas
ATI TEAS Exam

Describe the use of a pie chart.

Mathematics – Data Interpretation
© Mometrix Media - flashcardsecrets.com/teas
ATI TEAS Exam

Describe the use of a histogram.

Mathematics – Data Interpretation
© Mometrix Media - flashcardsecrets.com/teas
ATI TEAS Exam

Describe the use of a stem-and-leaf plot.

Mathematics – Data Interpretation
© Mometrix Media - flashcardsecrets.com/teas
ATI TEAS Exam

Describe the use of a scatter plot.

Mathematics – Data Interpretation
© Mometrix Media - flashcardsecrets.com/teas
ATI TEAS Exam

The following graph shows the ages of the five patients a nurse is caring for in the hospital:

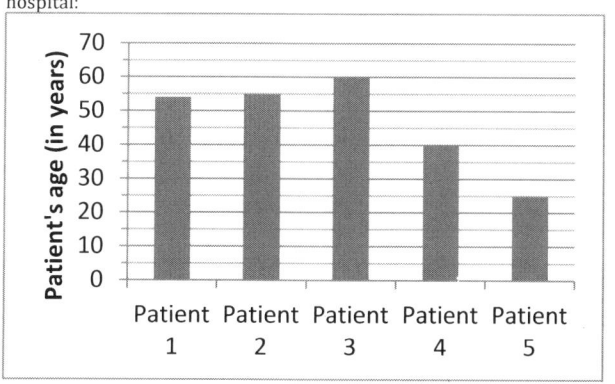

Use this graph to determine the age range of the patients for which the nurse is caring.

Mathematics – Data Interpretation
© Mometrix Media - flashcardsecrets.com/teas
ATI TEAS Exam

Below is a line graph representing the heart rate of a patient during the day. Use the graph to answer the questions that follow.

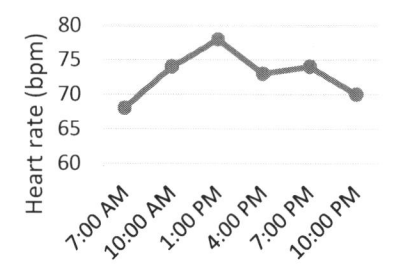

The patient's minimum measured heart rate occurred at what time? The patient's maximum measured heart rate occurred at what time? At what times during the day did the patient have the same measured heart rate?

A **histogram** is a special type of bar graph where the data are grouped in **intervals** (for example 20–29, 30–39, 40–49, etc.). The **frequency**, or number of times a value occurs in each interval, is indicated by the height of the bar. The intervals do not have to be the same amount but usually are (all data in ranges of 10 or all in ranges of 5, for example). The smaller the intervals, the more detailed the information.

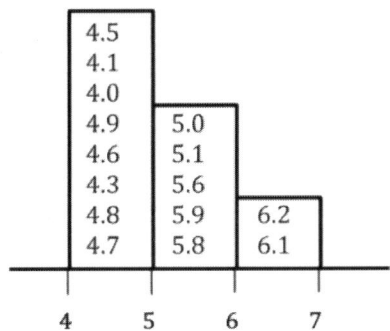

A **pie chart** or circle graph is a diagram used to compare parts of a whole. The full pie represents the whole, and it is divided into sectors that each represent something that is a part of the whole. Each sector or slice of the pie is either labeled to indicate what it represents, or explained on a key associated with the chart. The size of each slice is determined by the *percentage of the whole* that the associated quantity represents. Numerically, the angle measurement of each sector can be computed by solving the proportion: $x/360$ = part/whole.

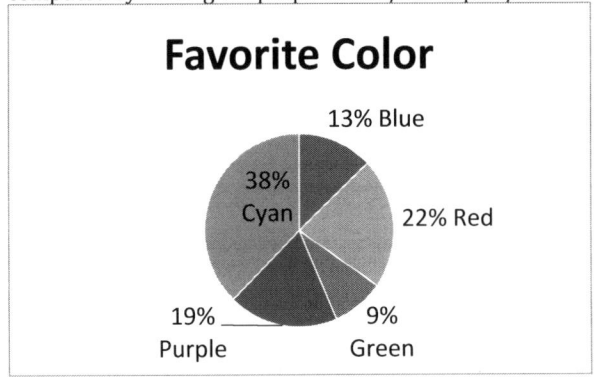

Scatter plots are useful for knowing the types of functions that are given with the data. Also, they are helpful for finding the simple regression. A **simple regression** is a regression that uses an independent variable.

A **regression** is a chart that is used to predict future events. Linear scatter plots may be positive or negative. Many nonlinear scatter plots are exponential or quadratic. Below are some common types of scatter plots:

A **stem-and-leaf plot** can outline groups of data that fall into a range of values. Each piece of data is split into two parts: the first, or left, part is called the stem. The second, or right, part is called the leaf. Each **stem** is listed in a column from smallest to largest. Each **leaf** that has the common stem is listed in that stem's row from smallest to largest.

For example, in a set of two-digit numbers, the digit in the tens place is the stem. So, the digit in the ones place is the leaf. With a stem-and-leaf plot, you can see which subset of numbers (10s, 20s, 30s, etc.) is the largest. This information can be found by looking at a histogram. However, a stem and leaf plot also lets you look closer and see which values fall in that range. Using all of the test scores from the line graph, we can put together a stem and leaf plot:

Test Scores									
7	4	8							
8	2	5	7	8	8				
9	0	0	1	2	2	3	5	8	9

Again, a stem-and-leaf plot is similar to histograms and frequency plots. However, a stem-and-leaf plot keeps all of the original data. In this example, you can see that almost half of the students scored in the 80s. Also, all of the data has been maintained. These plots can be used for larger numbers as well. However, they work better for *small sets of data*.

The patient's minimum measured heart rate occurred at the lowest data point on the graph, which is 68 bpm at 7:00 AM. The patient's maximum measured heart rate occurred at the highest data point on the graph, which is 78 bpm at 1:00 PM. The patient had the same measured heart rate of 74 bpm at 10:00 AM and 7:00 PM.

Use the graph to find the age of each patient: Patient 1 is 54 years old; Patient 2 is 55 years old; Patient 3 is 60 years old; Patient 4 is 40 years old; and Patient 5 is 25 years old. The age range is the age of the oldest patient minus the age of the youngest patient. In other words, 60 − 25 = 35. The age range is 35 years.

In a drug study containing 100 patients, a new cholesterol drug was found to decrease low-density lipoprotein (LDL) levels in 25% of the patients. In a second study containing 50 patients, the same drug administered at the same dosage was found to decrease LDL levels in 50% of the patients. Are the results of these two studies consistent with one another?

A nurse found the heart rates of eleven different patients to be 76, 80, 90, 86, 70, 76, 72, 88, 88, 68, and 88 beats per minute. Organize this information in a table.

Explain the term variable.

Ray earns $10 an hour at his job. Write an equation for his earnings as a function of time spent working. How long does Ray have to work in order to earn $360?

A patient told a doctor she feels fine after running one mile but that her knee starts hurting after running two miles. Her knee throbs after running three miles and swells after running four. Identify the independent and dependent variables with regard to the distance she runs and her level of pain.

Describe the term bivariate data.

There are several ways to organize data in a table. The table below is an example.

Patient Number	1	2	3	4	5	6
Heart Rate (bpm)	76	80	90	86	70	76
Patient Number	7	8	9	10	11	
Heart Rate (bpm)	72	88	88	68	88	

When making a table, be sure to label the columns and rows appropriately.

Even though in both studies 25 people (25% of 100 is 25 and 50% of 50 is 25) showed improvements in their LDL levels, the results of the studies are inconsistent. The results of the second study indicate that the drug has a much higher efficacy (desired result) than the results of the first study. Because 50 out of 150 total patients showed improvement on the medication, one could argue that the drug is effective in one third (or approximately 33%) of patients. However, one should be wary of the reliability of results when they're not **reproducible** from one study to the next and when the **sample size** is low.

The number of dollars that Ray earns is dependent on the number of hours he works, so earnings will be represented by the dependent variable y and hours worked will be represented by the independent variable x. He earns 10 dollars per hour worked, so his earning can be calculated as $y = 10x$.
To calculate the number of hours Ray must work in order to earn $360, plug in 360 for y and solve for x:

$$360 = 10x$$
$$x = \frac{360}{10} = 36$$

So, Ray must work 36 hours in order to earn $360.

A **variable** is a symbol, usually an alphabetic character, designating a *value that may change* within the scope of a given problem. Variables can be described as either independent or dependent variables. An **independent variable** is an input into a system that may take on values freely. **Dependent variables** are those that change as a consequence of changes in other values in the equation.

Bivariate data is data from two different variables. The prefix bi- means two. In a scatter plot, each value in the set of data is put on a grid. This is similar to the Cartesian plane where each axis represents one of the two variables. When you look at the pattern made by the points on the grid, you may know if there is a relationship between the two variables. Also, you may know what that relationship is and if it exists.
The variables may be directly proportionate, inversely proportionate, or show no proportion. Also, you may be able to see if the data is linear. If the data is linear, you can find an equation to show the two variables. The following scatter plot shows the relationship between preference for brand "A" and the age of the consumers surveyed.

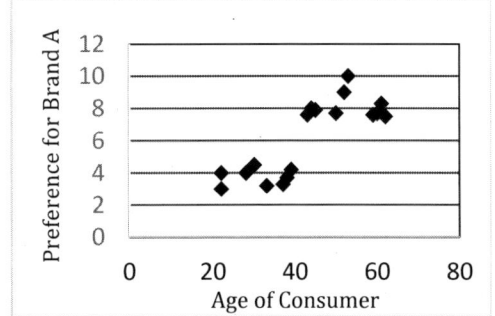

An independent variable is one that does not depend on any other variables in the situation. In this case, the distance the patient runs would be considered the independent variable. The dependent variable would be her level of pain because it depends on how far she runs.

Explain the term mean.

Explain the term median.

Explain the term mode.

Describe the term range.

Describe a skewed data set.

Describe unimodal and bimodal distribution.

The median is the value *in the middle of the data set*, in the sense that 50% of the data points lie above the median and 50% of the data points lie below. The median can be determined by simply putting the data points in order, and selecting the data point in the middle. If there is an even number of data points, then the median is the average of the middle two data points. For instance, for the data set {1, 3, 6, 8, 100, 800}, the median is $\frac{6+8}{2} = 7$.

For distributions with widely varying data points, especially those with large outliers, the median is a more appropriate measure of **central tendency**, and thus gives a better idea of a "typical" data point. Notice in the data set above, the mean is 153, while the median is 7.

The mean is the *average of the data points*; that is, it is the sum of the data points divided by the number of data points. Mathematically, the mean of a set of data points $\{x_1, x_2, x_3, \ldots x_n\}$ can be written as $\bar{X} = \sum \frac{X}{N}$. For instance, for the data set (1, 3, 6, 8, 100, 800), the mean is

$$\frac{1 + 3 + 6 + 8 + 100 + 800}{6} = 153$$

The mean is most useful when data is approximately normal and does not include extreme **outliers** (data values that are unusually high or unusually low compared to the rest of the data values). In the above example, the data shows much **variation**. Thus, the mean is not the best measure of central tendency to use, when interpreting the data. With this data set, the **median** will give a more complete picture of the distribution.

The range of a distribution is the *difference between the highest and lowest values in the distribution*. For example, in the data set (1, 3, 5, 7, 9, 11), the highest and lowest values are 11 and 1, respectively. The range then would be calculated as 11 – 1 = 10.

The mode is the value that *appears most often in the data set*. For instance, for the data set {2, 6, 4, 9, 4, 5, 7, 6, 4, 1, 5, 6, 7, 5, 6}, the mode is 6: the number 6 appears four times in the data set, while the next most frequent values, 4 and 5, appear only three times each. It is possible for a data set to have more than one mode: in the data set {11, 14, 17, 16, 11, 17, 12, 14, 17, 14, 13}, 14 and 17 are both modes, appearing three times each. In the extreme case of a uniform distribution—a distribution in which all values appear with equal probability—all values in the data set are modes. However, if no value appears more than once in a data set, the set has no mode.

The mode is useful to get a general sense of the *shape of the distribution*; it shows where the peaks of the distribution are. More information is necessary to get a more detailed description of the full shape.

If a distribution has a single peak, it would be considered **unimodal**. If it has two discernible peaks it would be considered **bimodal**. Bimodal distributions may be an indication that the set of data being considered is actually the combination of two sets of data with significant differences.

Symmetry is a characteristic of the shape of the plotted data. Specifically, it refers to how well the data on one side of the median *mirrors* the data on the other side.

A **skewed** data set is one that has a distinctly longer or fatter tail on one side of the peak or the other. A data set that is *skewed left* has more of its values to the left of the peak, while a set that is *skewed right* has more of its values to the right of the peak. When actually looking at the graph, these names may seem counterintuitive since, in a left-skewed data set, the bulk of the values seem to be on the right side of the graph, and vice versa. However, if the graph is viewed strictly in relation to the peak, the direction of skewness makes more sense.

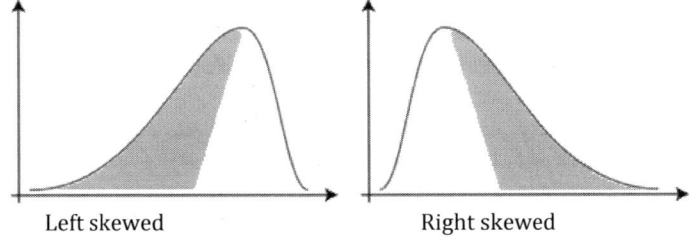

Mathematics – Data Interpretation
© Mometrix Media - flashcardsecrets.com/teas
ATI TEAS Exam

Describe uniform distribution.

Mathematics – Measurement
© Mometrix Media - flashcardsecrets.com/teas
ATI TEAS Exam

Describe a quadrilateral and parallelogram.

Mathematics – Measurement
© Mometrix Media - flashcardsecrets.com/teas
ATI TEAS Exam

Describe a trapezoid.

Mathematics – Measurement
© Mometrix Media - flashcardsecrets.com/teas
ATI TEAS Exam

Describe a rectangle, square, and rhombus.

Mathematics – Measurement
© Mometrix Media - flashcardsecrets.com/teas
ATI TEAS Exam

Describe the different types of quadrilaterals.

Mathematics – Measurement
© Mometrix Media - flashcardsecrets.com/teas
ATI TEAS Exam

Explain the center, radius, and diameter of a circle.

Quadrilateral: A closed two-dimensional geometric figure composed of exactly four straight sides. The sum of the interior angles of any quadrilateral is 360°.

Parallelogram: A quadrilateral that has exactly two pairs of opposite **parallel** sides. The sides that are parallel are also **congruent**. The opposite interior angles are always congruent, and the consecutive interior angles are **supplementary**. The **diagonals** of a parallelogram bisect each other. Each diagonal divides the parallelogram into two congruent triangles.

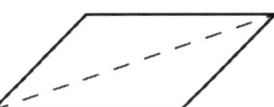

A **uniform** distribution is a distribution in which there is *no distinct peak or variation* in the data. No values or ranges are particularly more common than any other values or ranges.

Rectangle: A parallelogram with four right angles. All rectangles are parallelograms, but not all parallelograms are rectangles. The diagonals of a rectangle are congruent.

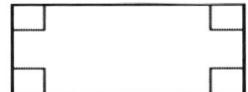

Rhombus: A parallelogram with four congruent sides. All rhombuses are parallelograms, but not all parallelograms are rhombuses. The diagonals of a rhombus are **perpendicular** to each other.

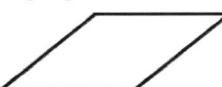

Square: A parallelogram with four right angles and four congruent sides. All squares are also parallelograms, rhombuses, and rectangles. The diagonals of a square are congruent and perpendicular to each other.

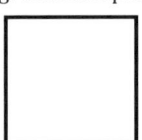

Trapezoid: Traditionally, a quadrilateral that has exactly one pair of parallel sides. Some math texts define trapezoid as a quadrilateral that has at least one pair of parallel sides. Because there are no rules governing the second pair of sides, there are no rules that apply to the properties of the diagonals of a trapezoid.

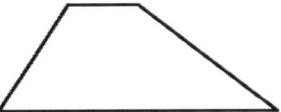

The **center** is the single point inside the circle that is **equidistant** from every point on the circle. (Point *O* in the diagram below.)

The **radius** is a line segment that joins the center of the circle and any one point on the circle. All radii of a circle are equal. (Segments *OX*, *OY*, and *OZ* in the diagram below.)

The **diameter** is a line segment that passes through the center of the circle and has both endpoints on the circle. The length of the diameter is exactly *twice the length of the radius*. (Segment *XZ* in the diagram below.)

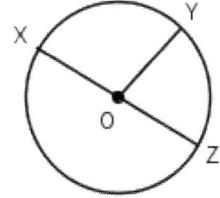

A quadrilateral whose diagonals bisect each other is a **parallelogram**. A quadrilateral whose opposite sides are parallel (2 pairs of parallel sides) is a parallelogram.

A quadrilateral whose diagonals are perpendicular bisectors is a **rhombus**. A quadrilateral whose opposite sides (both pairs) are parallel and congruent is a rhombus.

A parallelogram that has a right angle is a **rectangle**. (Consecutive angles of a parallelogram are supplementary. Therefore, if there is one right angle in a parallelogram, there are four right angles in that parallelogram.)

A rhombus that has a right angle is a **square**. Because the rhombus is a special form of a parallelogram, the rules about the angles of a parallelogram also apply to the rhombus.

Describe an arc, central angle, minor arc, and semicircle.

Describe a chord and secant.

Describe an inscribed angle.

Explain the arc length on a circle.

Describe a sector on a circle.

Explain how to find the perimeter of a triangle.

A **chord** is a line segment that has both endpoints on a circle. In the diagram below, $\overline{EB}$ is a chord.

Secant: A line that passes through a circle and contains a chord of that circle. In the diagram below, $\overleftrightarrow{EB}$ is a secant and contains chord $\overline{EB}$.

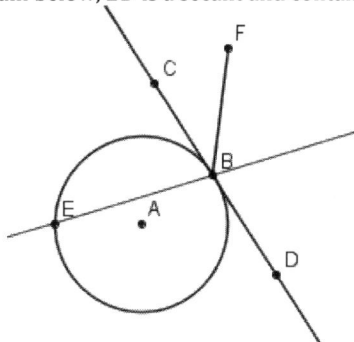

An **arc** is a portion of a circle. Specifically, an arc is the set of points between and including two points on a circle. An arc does not contain any points inside the circle. When a segment is drawn from the endpoints of an arc to the center of the circle, a **sector** is formed.

A **central angle** is an angle whose **vertex** is the center of a circle and whose legs intercept an arc of the circle. Angle *XOY* in the diagram above is a central angle. A **minor arc** is an arc that has a measure less than 180°. The measure of a central angle is equal to the measure of the minor arc it intercepts. A **major arc** is an arc having a measure of at least 180°. The measure of the major arc can be found by subtracting the measure of the central angle from 360°.

A **semicircle** is an arc whose endpoints are the endpoints of the diameter of a circle. A semicircle is exactly half of a circle.

The **arc length** is the length of that portion of the circumference between two points on the circle. The formula for arc length is $s = \frac{\pi r \theta}{180°}$ where *s* is the arc length, *r* is the length of the radius, and θ is the angular measure of the arc in degrees, or $s = r\theta$, where θ is the angular measure of the arc in radians (2π radians = 360 degrees).

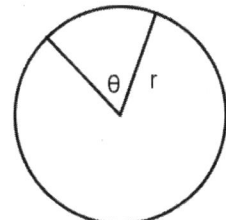

An **inscribed angle** is an angle whose vertex lies on a circle and whose legs contain chords of that circle. The portion of the circle intercepted by the legs of the angle is called the **intercepted arc**. The measure of the intercepted arc is exactly twice the measure of the inscribed angle. In the diagram below, angle *ABC* is an inscribed angle. $\widehat{AC} = 2(m\angle ABC)$.

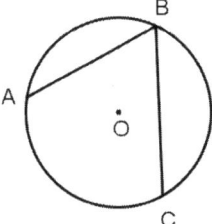

The **perimeter** of any triangle is found by summing the three side lengths; $P = a + b + c$. For an **equilateral triangle**, this is the same as $P = 3s$, where *s* is any side length, since all three sides are the same length.

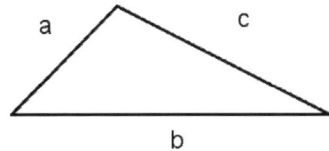

A **sector** is the portion of a circle formed by two radii and their intercepted arc. While the arc length is exclusively the points that are also on the circumference of the circle, the sector is the entire area bounded by the arc and the two radii.

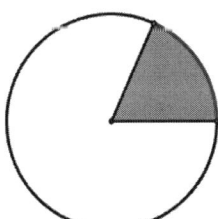

The **area** of a sector of a circle is found by the formula $A = \frac{\theta r^2}{2}$, where *A* is the area, θ is the measure of the central angle in radians, and *r* is the radius. To find the area when the central angle is in degrees, use the formula, $A = \frac{\theta \pi r^2}{360}$, where θ is the measure of the central angle in degrees and *r* is the radius.

Mathematics – Measurement
© Mometrix Media - flashcardsecrets.com/teas
ATI TEAS Exam

Explain how to find the perimeter of a square, rectangle, and parallelogram.

Mathematics – Measurement
© Mometrix Media - flashcardsecrets.com/teas
ATI TEAS Exam

Explain how to find the perimeter of a trapezoid.

Mathematics – Measurement
© Mometrix Media - flashcardsecrets.com/teas
ATI TEAS Exam

Explain how to find the area of a triangle, square, and rectangle.

Mathematics – Measurement
© Mometrix Media - flashcardsecrets.com/teas
ATI TEAS Exam

Explain how to find the area of a parallelogram, trapezoid, and a circle.

Mathematics – Measurement
© Mometrix Media - flashcardsecrets.com/teas
ATI TEAS Exam

Describe base surface area and lateral surface area.

Mathematics – Measurement
© Mometrix Media - flashcardsecrets.com/teas
ATI TEAS Exam

Describe how to find the surface area of a prism.

Visit *mometrix.com/academy* for a related video.
Enter video code: 163343

Trapezoid
The perimeter of a trapezoid is found by the formula $P = a + b_1 + c + b_2$, where a, b_1, c, and b_2 are the four sides of the trapezoid.

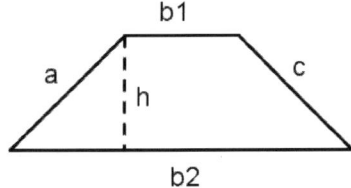

Circle
The perimeter (**circumference**) of a circle is found by the formula $C = 2\pi r$, where r is the radius. Again, remember to convert the diameter if you are given that measure rather than the radius.

Square
The perimeter of a square is found by using the formula $P = 4s$, where s is the length of one side. Because all four sides are equal in a square, it is faster to multiply the length of one side by 4 than to add the same number four times. You could use the formulas for rectangles and get the same answer.

Rectangle
The perimeter of a rectangle is found by the formula $P = 2l + 2w$ or $P = 2(l + w)$, where l is the length, and w is the width. It may be easier to add the length and width first and then double the result, as in the second formula.

Parallelogram
The perimeter of a parallelogram is found by the formula $P = 2a + 2b$ or $P = 2(a + b)$, where a and b are the lengths of the two sides.

Parallelogram
The area of a parallelogram is found by the formula $A = bh$, where b is the length of the base and h is the height. Note that the base and height correspond to the length and width in a rectangle, so this formula would apply to rectangles as well. Do not confuse the height of a parallelogram with the length of the second side. The two are only the same measure in the case of a rectangle.

Trapezoid
The area of a trapezoid is found by the formula $A = \frac{1}{2}h(b_1 + b_2)$, where h is the height (segment joining and perpendicular to the parallel bases), and b_1 and b_2 are the two parallel sides (bases). Do not use one of the other two sides as the height unless that side is also perpendicular to the parallel bases.

Circle
The area of a circle is found by the formula $A = \pi r^2$, where r is the length of the radius. If the diameter of the circle is given, remember to divide it in half to get the length of the radius before proceeding.

Triangle
The **area** of any triangle can be found by taking half the product of one side length (base or b) and the perpendicular distance from that side to the opposite vertex (height or h). In equation form, $A = \frac{1}{2}bh$.

Square
The area of a square is found by using the formula $A = s^2$, where and s is the length of one side.

Rectangle
The area of a rectangle is found by the formula $A = lw$, where A is the area of the rectangle, l is the length (usually considered to be the longer side) and w is the width (usually considered to be the shorter side). The numbers for l and w are interchangeable.

The **surface area** of any prism is the sum of the areas of both bases and all sides. It can be calculated as $SA = 2B + Ph$, where P is the perimeter of the base. The **volume** of any prism is found with the formula $V = Bh$, where B is the area of the base and h is the height. The perpendicular distance between the bases is the height.

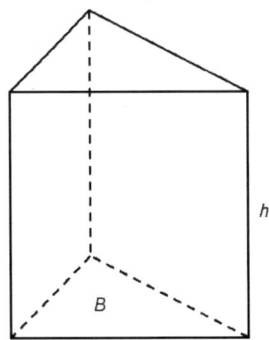

The surface area of a solid object is the *area of all sides or exterior surfaces*. For objects such as prisms and pyramids, a further distinction is made between **base surface area** (B) and **lateral surface area** (LA). For a prism, the total surface area (SA) is $SA = LA + 2B$. For a pyramid or cone, the total surface area is $SA = LA + B$.

Mathematics – Measurement
ATI TEAS Exam

Describe how to find the surface area of a sphere.

Mathematics – Measurement
ATI TEAS Exam

Dwight has a beach ball with a radius of 9 inches. He is planning to wrap the ball with wrapping paper. How many square feet of wrapping paper are needed to cover the surface of the ball?

Mathematics – Measurement
ATI TEAS Exam

Describe how to find the surface area and volume of a cube.

Mathematics – Measurement
ATI TEAS Exam

Describe how to find the surface area and volume of a rectangular prism.

Mathematics – Measurement
ATI TEAS Exam

Describe how to find the surface area and volume of a cylinder.

Mathematics – Measurement
ATI TEAS Exam

Describe how a Cartesian coordinate plane is used.

The surface area of a sphere may be calculated using the formula $SA = 4\pi r^2$. Substituting 9 for r gives $SA = 4\pi(9)^2$, which simplifies to $SA \approx 1017.36$. So the surface area of the ball is approximately 1017.36 square inches. There are twelve inches in a foot. So, there are $12^2 = 144$ square inches in a square foot. To convert this measurement to square feet, the following proportion may be written and solved for x: $\frac{1}{144} = \frac{x}{1017.36}$. So $x \approx 7.07$, meaning it will take approximately 7.07 square feet of wrapping paper to cover the surface of the ball.

The **surface area** of a sphere can be found by the formula $A = 4\pi r^2$, where r is the radius. The **volume** of a sphere can be found with the formula $V = \frac{4}{3}\pi r^3$, where r is the radius. Both quantities are generally given in terms of π.

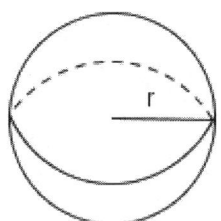

The **surface area** can be calculated as $SA = 2lw + 2hl + 2wh$ or $SA = 2(lw + hl + wh)$. The **volume** of a rectangular prism can be found with the formula $V = lwh$, where V is the volume, l is the length, w is the width, and h is the height.

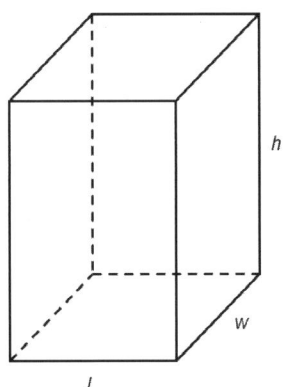

The **volume** of a cube can be found with the formula $V = s^3$, where s is the length of a side.

The **surface area** of a cube is calculated as $SA = 6s^2$, where SA is the total surface area and s is the length of a side. These formulas are the same as the ones used for the volume and surface area of a rectangular prism. However, these are simple formulas because the three numbers (i.e., length, width, and height) are the same.

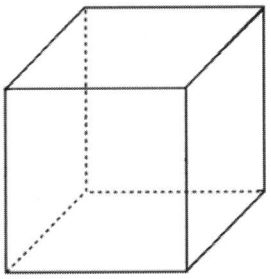

When algebraic functions and equations are shown graphically, they are usually shown on a **Cartesian coordinate plane**. The Cartesian coordinate plane consists of two number lines placed perpendicular to each other, and intersecting at the **zero point**, also known as the **origin**. The horizontal number line is known as the **x-axis**, with positive values to the right of the origin and negative values to the left of the origin. The vertical number line is known as the **y-axis**, with positive values above the origin and negative values below the origin. Any point on the plane can be identified by an ordered pair in the form (x,y), called **coordinates**. The x-value of the coordinate is called the **abscissa**, and the y-value of the coordinate is called the **ordinate**. The two number lines divide the plane into four **quadrants**: I, II, III, and IV.

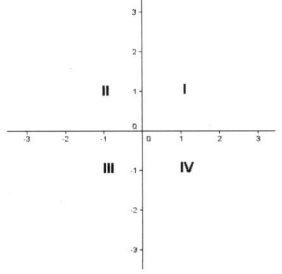

The **surface area** of a cylinder can be found by the formula $SA = 2\pi r^2 + 2\pi rh$. The first term is the base area multiplied by two, and the second term is the perimeter of the base multiplied by the height. The **volume** of a cylinder can be found with the formula $V = \pi r^2 h$, where r is the radius and h is the height.

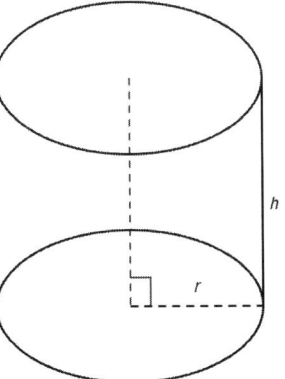

Mathematics – Measurement
© Mometrix Media - flashcardsecrets.com/teas
ATI TEAS Exam

Plot the following points on the coordinate plane:
A. (–4, –2) B. (–1, 3)   C. (2, 2)   D. (3, –1)

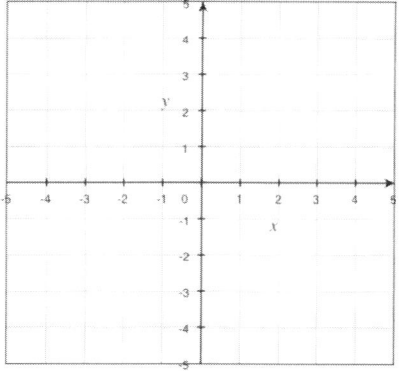

Mathematics – Measurement
© Mometrix Media - flashcardsecrets.com/teas
ATI TEAS Exam

A map has a key for measurements to compare real distances with a scale distance.
The key on one map says that 2 inches on the map is 12 real miles. Find the distance of a route that is 5 inches long on the map.

Mathematics – Measurement
© Mometrix Media - flashcardsecrets.com/teas
ATI TEAS Exam

Describe the process of going from a larger unit to a smaller unit.

Visit *mometrix.com/academy* for a related video.
Enter video code: 163709

Mathematics – Measurement
© Mometrix Media - flashcardsecrets.com/teas
ATI TEAS Exam

Describe metric conversions.

Mathematics – Measurement
© Mometrix Media - flashcardsecrets.com/teas
ATI TEAS Exam

Describe U.S. and metric equivalents.

Mathematics – Measurement
© Mometrix Media - flashcardsecrets.com/teas
ATI TEAS Exam

Describe capacity measurements.

A **proportion** is needed to show the map measurements and real distances. First, write a ratio that has the information in the key. The map measurement can be in the numerator, and the real distance can be in the denominator.

$$\frac{2 \text{ inches}}{12 \text{ miles}}$$

Next, write a ratio with the known map distance and the unknown real distance. The unknown number for miles can be represented with the letter *m*.

$$\frac{5 \text{ inches}}{m \text{ miles}}$$

Then, write out the ratios in a proportion and solve it for *m*.

$$\frac{2 \text{ inches}}{12 \text{ miles}} = \frac{5 \text{ inches}}{m \text{ miles}}$$

Now, you have $2m = 60$. So, you are left with $m = 30$. Thus, the route is 30 miles long.

Answer:

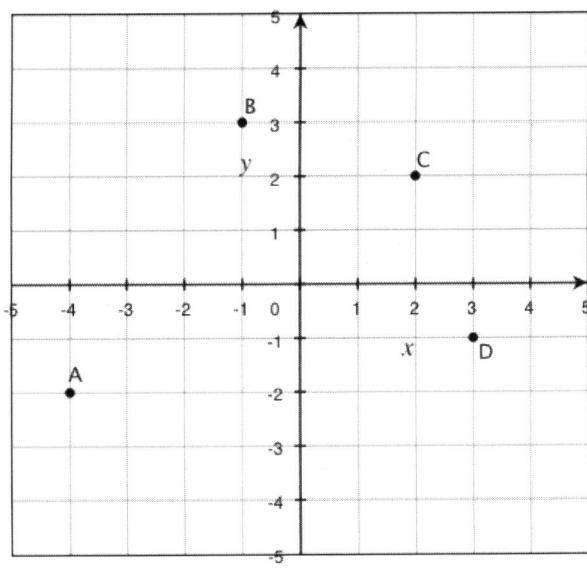

Metric Conversions

1000 mcg (microgram)	1 mg
1000 mg (milligram)	1 g
1000 g (gram)	1 kg
1000 kg (kilogram)	1 metric ton
1000 mL (milliliter)	1 L
1000 um (micrometer)	1 mm
1000 mm (millimeter)	1 m
100 cm (centimeter)	1 m
1000 m (meter)	1 km

When going from a larger unit to a smaller unit, multiply the number of the known amount by the **equivalent amount**. When going from a smaller unit to a larger unit, divide the number of the known amount by the equivalent amount.

Also, you can set up conversion fractions. In these fractions, one fraction is the **conversion factor**. The other fraction has the unknown amount in the numerator. So, the known value is placed in the denominator. Sometimes the second fraction has the known value from the problem in the numerator, and the unknown in the denominator. Multiply the two fractions to get the converted measurement.

Capacity Measurements

Unit	U.S. equivalent	Metric equivalent
Ounce	8 drams	29.573 milliliters
Cup	8 ounces	0.237 liter
Pint	16 ounces	0.473 liter
Quart	2 pints	0.946 liter
Gallon	4 quarts	3.785 liters

U.S. and Metric Equivalents

Unit	U.S. equivalent	Metric equivalent
Inch	1 inch	2.54 centimeters
Foot	12 inches	0.305 meters
Yard	3 feet	0.914 meters
Mile	5280 feet	1.609 kilometers

Mathematics – Measurement
© Mometrix Media - flashcardsecrets.com/teas
ATI TEAS Exam

Describe weight measurements and nursing measurements.

Visit *mometrix.com/academy* for a related video.
Enter video code: 241463

Mathematics – Measurement
© Mometrix Media - flashcardsecrets.com/teas
ATI TEAS Exam

a. Convert 1.4 meters to centimeters.
b. Convert 218 centimeters to meters.

Mathematics – Measurement
© Mometrix Media - flashcardsecrets.com/teas
ATI TEAS Exam

a. Convert 42 inches to feet.
b. Convert 15 feet to yards.

Mathematics – Measurement
© Mometrix Media - flashcardsecrets.com/teas
ATI TEAS Exam

a. How many pounds are in 15 kilograms?
b. How many pounds are in 80 ounces?

Mathematics – Measurement
© Mometrix Media - flashcardsecrets.com/teas
ATI TEAS Exam

a. How many kilometers are in 2 miles?
b. How many centimeters are in 5 feet?

Mathematics – Measurement
© Mometrix Media - flashcardsecrets.com/teas
ATI TEAS Exam

a. How many gallons are in 15.14 liters?
b. How many liters are in 8 quarts?

Write ratios with the conversion factor $\frac{100 \text{ cm}}{1 \text{ m}}$. Use proportions to convert the given units.

a. $\frac{100 \text{ cm}}{1 \text{ m}} = \frac{x \text{ cm}}{1.4 \text{ m}}$. Cross multiply to get $x = 140$. So, 1.4 m is the same as 140 cm.

b. $\frac{100 \text{ cm}}{1 \text{ m}} = \frac{218 \text{ cm}}{x \text{ m}}$. Cross multiply to get $100x = 218$, or $x = 2.18$. So, 218 cm is the same as 2.18 m.

Weight Measurements

Unit	U.S. equivalent	Metric equivalent
Ounce	16 drams	28.35 grams
Pound	16 ounces	453.6 grams
Ton	2,000 pounds	907.2 kilograms

Nursing Measurements

Unit	English equivalent	Metric equivalent
1 tsp	1.333 fluid dram	5 milliliters
3 tsp	4 fluid drams	15 or 16 milliliters
2 tbsp	1 fluid ounce	30 milliliters
1 glass	8 fluid ounces	240 milliliters

a. 15 kilograms $\times \frac{2.2 \text{ pounds}}{1 \text{ kilogram}} = 33$ pounds

b. 80 ounces $\times \frac{1 \text{ pound}}{16 \text{ ounces}} = 5$ pounds

Write ratios with the conversion factors $\frac{12 \text{ in}}{1 \text{ ft}}$ and $\frac{3 \text{ ft}}{1 \text{ yd}}$. Use proportions to convert the given units.

a. $\frac{12 \text{ in}}{1 \text{ ft}} = \frac{42 \text{ in}}{x \text{ ft}}$. Cross multiply to get $12x = 42$, or $x = 3.5$. So, 42 inches is the same as 3.5 feet.

b. $\frac{3 \text{ ft}}{1 \text{ yd}} = \frac{15 \text{ ft}}{x \text{ yd}}$. Cross multiply to get $3x = 15$, or $x = 5$. So, 15 feet is the same as 5 yards.

a. 15.14 liters $\times \frac{1 \text{ gallon}}{3.785 \text{ liters}} = 4$ gallons

b. 8 quarts $\times \frac{1 \text{ gallon}}{4 \text{ quarts}} \times \frac{3.785 \text{ liters}}{1 \text{ gallon}} = 7.57$ liters

a. 2 miles $\times \frac{1.609 \text{ kilometers}}{1 \text{ mile}} = 3.218$ kilometers

b. 5 feet $\times \frac{12 \text{ inches}}{1 \text{ foot}} \times \frac{2.54 \text{ centimeters}}{1 \text{ inch}} = 152.4$ centimeters

Mathematics – Measurement
© Mometrix Media - flashcardsecrets.com/teas
ATI TEAS Exam

a. How many grams are in 13.2 pounds?
b. How many pints are in 9 gallons?

Science – Human Anatomy and Physiology
© Mometrix Media - flashcardsecrets.com/teas
ATI TEAS Exam

Explain the role of a cell and describe its basic contents.

Science – Human Anatomy and Physiology
© Mometrix Media - flashcardsecrets.com/teas
ATI TEAS Exam

Describe structural organization of organisms.

Science – Human Anatomy and Physiology
© Mometrix Media - flashcardsecrets.com/teas
ATI TEAS Exam

Define and describe the following nuclear parts of a eukaryotic cell: nucleus, chromosomes, chromatin, nucleolus, nuclear envelope, nuclear pores, and nucleoplasm.

Science – Human Anatomy and Physiology
© Mometrix Media - flashcardsecrets.com/teas
ATI TEAS Exam

Describe the structure and function of cell membranes.

Science – Human Anatomy and Physiology
© Mometrix Media - flashcardsecrets.com/teas
ATI TEAS Exam

Describe how cells use selective permeability to maintain their internal environment and respond to external signs.

The cell is the basic *organizational unit* of all living things. Each piece within a cell has a function that helps organisms grow and survive. There are many different types of cells, but cells are unique to each type of organism. The one thing that all cells have in common is a **membrane**, which is comparable to a semi-permeable plastic bag. The membrane is composed of **phospholipids**. There are also some **transport holes**, which are proteins that help certain molecules and ions move in and out of the cell. The cell is filled with a fluid called **cytoplasm** or cytosol. Within the cell are a variety of **organelles**, groups of complex molecules that help a cell survive, each with its own unique membrane that has a different chemical makeup from the cell membrane. The larger the cell, the more organelles it will need to live.

a. $13.2 \text{ pounds} \times \frac{1 \text{ kilogram}}{2.2 \text{ pounds}} \times \frac{1000 \text{ grams}}{1 \text{ kilogram}} = 6000 \text{ grams}$

b. $9 \text{ gallons} \times \frac{4 \text{ quarts}}{1 \text{ gallon}} \times \frac{2 \text{ pints}}{1 \text{ quarts}} = 72 \text{ pints}$

- **Nucleus** (pl. nuclei): This is a small structure that contains the **chromosomes** and regulates the **DNA** of a cell. The nucleus is the defining structure of **eukaryotic cells**, and all eukaryotic cells have a nucleus. The nucleus is responsible for the passing on of genetic traits between generations. The nucleus contains a *nuclear envelope, nucleoplasm, a nucleolus, nuclear pores, chromatin, and ribosomes.*
- **Chromosomes**: These are highly condensed, threadlike rods of DNA. Short for **deoxyribonucleic acid**, DNA is the genetic material that *stores information about the plant or animal.*
- **Chromatin**: This consists of the DNA and protein that make up **chromosomes**.
- **Nucleolus**: This structure contained within the nucleus consists of protein. It is small, round, does not have a membrane, is involved in **protein synthesis**, and synthesizes and stores **RNA (ribonucleic acid)**.
- **Nuclear envelope**: This encloses the structures of the nucleus. It consists of inner and outer membranes made of **lipids**.
- **Nuclear pores**: These are involved in the exchange of material between the nucleus and the **cytoplasm**.
- **Nucleoplasm**: This is the liquid within the nucleus, and is similar to cytoplasm.

All organisms, whether plants, animals, fungi, protists, or bacteria, exhibit structural organization on the cellular and organism level. All cells contain **DNA** and **RNA** and can synthesize proteins. All organisms have a highly organized cellular structure. Each cell consists of **nucleic acids**, **cytoplasm**, and a **cell membrane**. Specialized organelles such as **mitochondria** and **chloroplasts** have specific functions within the cell. In single-celled organisms, that single cell contains all of the components necessary for life. In multicellular organisms, cells can become specialized. Different types of cells can have different functions. Life begins as a single cell whether by **asexual** or **sexual reproduction**. Cells are grouped together in **tissues**. Tissues are grouped together in **organs**. Organs are grouped together in **systems**. An **organism** is a complete individual.

The cell membrane, or plasma membrane, has **selective permeability** with regard to size, charge, and solubility. With regard to molecule size, the cell membrane allows only small molecules to diffuse through it. **Oxygen** and **water** molecules are small and typically can pass through the cell membrane. The charge of the **ions** on the cell's surface also either attracts or repels ions. Ions with like charges are repelled, and ions with opposite charges are attracted to the cell's surface. Molecules that are soluble in **phospholipids** can usually pass through the cell membrane. Many molecules are not able to diffuse the cell membrane, and, if needed, those molecules must be moved through by active transport and **vesicles**.

The cell membrane, also referred to as the **plasma membrane**, is a thin semipermeable membrane of lipids and proteins. The cell membrane isolates the cell from its external environment while still enabling the cell to communicate with that outside environment. It consists of a **phospholipid bilayer**, or double layer, with the **hydrophilic ends** of the outer layer facing the external environment, the inner layer facing the inside of the cell, and the **hydrophobic ends** facing each other. **Cholesterol** in the cell membrane adds stiffness and flexibility. **Glycolipids** help the cell to recognize other cells of the organisms. The **proteins** in the cell membrane help give the cells shape. Special proteins help the cell communicate with its external environment. Other proteins transport molecules across the cell membrane.

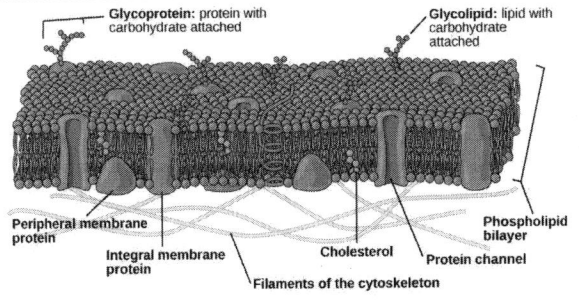

Define and describe the following cell structures: ribosomes, Golgi complex, vacuoles, vesicle, cytoskeleton, and microtubules.

Define and describe the following cell structures: cytosol, cytoplasm, cell membrane, endoplasmic reticulum, and mitochondrion.

Describe the four functions of the mitochondria.

Define and describe the following structures that are unique to animal cells: centrosome, centriole, lysosome, cilia, and flagella.

Define and discuss the cell cycle.

Discuss cell differentiation.

Cytosol: This is the *liquid material in the cell*. It is mostly water, but also contains some floating molecules.

Cytoplasm: This is a general term that refers to cytosol and the substructures (organelles) found *within the plasma membrane*, but not within the nucleus.

Cell membrane (plasma membrane): This defines the cell by acting as a *barrier*. It helps keeps cytoplasm in and substances located outside the cell out. It also determines what is allowed to enter and exit the cell.

Endoplasmic reticulum: The two types of endoplasmic reticulum are **rough** (has ribosomes on the surface) and **smooth** (does not have ribosomes on the surface). It is a tubular network that comprises the *transport system of a cell*. It is fused to the nuclear membrane and extends through the cytoplasm to the cell membrane.

Mitochondrion (pl. mitochondria): These cell structures vary in terms of size and quantity. Some cells may have one mitochondrion, while others have thousands. This structure performs various functions such as *generating ATP*, and is also involved in *cell growth and death*. Mitochondria contain their own DNA that is separate from that contained in the nucleus.

Ribosomes: Ribosomes are involved in *synthesizing proteins from amino acids*. They are numerous, making up about one quarter of the cell. Some cells contain thousands of ribosomes. Some are mobile and some are embedded in the rough **endoplasmic reticulum**.

Golgi complex (Golgi apparatus): This is involved in *synthesizing materials* such as proteins that are transported out of the cell. It is located near the nucleus and consists of layers of **membranes**.

Vacuoles: These are sacs used for *storage, digestion, and waste removal*. There is one large vacuole in plant cells. Animal cells have small, sometimes numerous vacuoles.

Vesicle: This is a small organelle within a cell. It has a membrane and performs varying functions, including *moving materials within a cell*.

Cytoskeleton: This consists of **microtubules** that help *shape and support the cell*.

Microtubules: These are part of the **cytoskeleton** and help *support the cell*. They are made of protein.

Centrosome: This is comprised of the pair of **centrioles** located at right angles to each other and surrounded by protein. The centrosome is involved in *mitosis and the cell cycle*.

Centrioles: These are cylinder-shaped structures near the nucleus that are involved in *cellular division*. Each cylinder consists of nine groups of three **microtubules**. Centrioles occur in pairs.

Lysosome: This *digests proteins, lipids, and carbohydrates*, and also *transports undigested substances* to the cell membrane so they can be removed. The shape of a lysosome depends on the material being transported.

Cilia (singular: cilium): These are appendages extending from the surface of the cell, the movement of which *causes the cell to move*. They can also result in fluid being moved by the cell.

Flagella: These are tail-like structures on cells that use whip-like movements to *help the cell move*. They are similar to cilia, but are usually longer and not as numerous. A cell usually only has one or a few flagella.

Four functions of mitochondria are: the production of **cell energy**, **cell signaling** (how communications are carried out within a cell, **cellular differentiation** (the process whereby a non-differentiated cell becomes transformed into a cell with a more specialized purpose), and **cell cycle and growth regulation** (the process whereby the cell gets ready to reproduce and reproduces). Mitochondria are numerous in eukaryotic cells. There may be hundreds or even thousands of mitochondria in a single cell. Mitochondria can be involved in many functions, their main one being *supplying the cell with energy*. Mitochondria consist of an inner and outer membrane. The inner membrane encloses the **matrix**, which contains the **mitochondrial DNA** (mtDNA) and ribosomes. Between the inner and outer membranes are **folds** (cristae). Chemical reactions occur here that release energy, control water levels in cells, and recycle and create proteins and fats. **Aerobic respiration** also occurs in the mitochondria.

The human body is filled with many different types of cells. The process that helps to determine the cell type for each cell is known as **differentiation**. Another way to say this is when *a less-specialized cell becomes a more-specialized cell*. This process is controlled by the genes of each cell among a group of cells known as *a zygote*. Following the directions of the genes, a cell builds certain proteins and other pieces that set it apart as a specific type of cell.

An example occurs with **gastrulation**—an early phase in the embryonic development of most animals. During gastrulation, the cells are organized into three primary germ layers: **ectoderm, mesoderm**, and **endoderm**. Then, the cells in these layers differentiate into special tissues and organs. For example, the *nervous system* develops from the ectoderm. The *muscular system* develops from the mesoderm. Much of the *digestive system* develops from the endoderm.

The term cell cycle refers to the process by which a cell **reproduces**, which involves *cell growth, the duplication of genetic material, and cell division*. Complex organisms with many cells use the cell cycle to replace cells as they lose their functionality and wear out. The entire cell cycle in animal cells can take 24 hours. The time required varies among different cell types. Human skin cells, for example, are constantly reproducing. Some other cells only divide infrequently. Once neurons are mature, they do not grow or divide. The two ways that cells can reproduce are through meiosis and mitosis. When cells replicate through **mitosis**, the "daughter cell" is an *exact replica* of the parent cell. When cells divide through **meiosis**, the daughter cells have *different genetic coding* than the parent cell. Meiosis only happens in specialized reproductive cells called **gametes**.

List the primary events that occur during mitosis.

Visit *mometrix.com/academy* for a related video.
Enter video code: 894894

List the primary events that occur during meiosis.

List and define the seven categories of animal tissues.

Describe the functions of organs.

List the three primary body planes.

Define the terms medial, lateral, proximal, distal, anterior, and posterior.

Meiosis has the same phases as mitosis, but they happen twice. In addition, different events occur during some phases of meiosis than mitosis. The events that occur during the first phase of meiosis are interphase (I), prophase (I), metaphase (I), anaphase (I), telophase (I), and cytokinesis (I). During this first phase of meiosis, *chromosomes cross over, genetic material is exchanged, and tetrads of four chromatids are formed.* The nuclear membrane dissolves. Homologous pairs of chromatids are separated and travel to different poles. At this point, there has been one cell division resulting in two cells. Each cell goes through a second cell division, which consists of prophase (II), metaphase (II), anaphase (II), telophase (II), and cytokinesis (II). The result is *four daughter cells* with different sets of chromosomes. The daughter cells are **haploid**, which means they contain half the genetic material of the parent cell. The second phase of meiosis is similar to the process of mitosis. Meiosis encourages genetic diversity.

The primary events that occur during mitosis are:
- **Interphase**: The cell prepares for division by replicating its genetic and cytoplasmic material. Interphase can be further divided into G_1, S, and G_2.
- **Prophase**: The **chromatin** thickens into chromosomes and the **nuclear membrane** begins to disintegrate. Pairs of **centrioles** move to opposite sides of the cell and spindle fibers begin to form. The **mitotic spindle**, formed from cytoskeleton parts, moves chromosomes around within the cell.
- **Metaphase**: The spindle moves to the center of the cell and chromosome pairs align along the center of the spindle structure.
- **Anaphase**: The pairs of chromosomes, called sisters, begin to pull apart, and may bend. When they are separated, they are called **daughter chromosomes**. Grooves appear in the cell membrane.
- **Telophase**: The spindle disintegrates, the nuclear membranes reform, and the chromosomes revert to chromatin. In animal cells, the membrane is pinched. In plant cells, a new cell wall begins to form.
- **Cytokinesis**: This is the physical splitting of the cell (including the cytoplasm) into two cells. Some believe this occurs following telophase. Others say it occurs from anaphase, as the cell begins to furrow, through telophase, when the cell actually splits into two.

Organs are groups of tissues that work together to perform specific functions. Complex animals have several organs that are grouped together in multiple **systems**. For example, the **heart** is specifically designed to pump blood throughout an organism's body. The heart is composed mostly of muscle tissue in the myocardium, but it also contains connective tissue in the blood and membranes, nervous tissue that controls the heart rate, and epithelial tissue in the membranes. Gills in fish and lungs in reptiles, birds, and mammals are specifically designed to exchange gases. In birds, crops are designed to store food and gizzards are designed to grind food.

Organ systems are groups of organs that work together to perform specific functions. In mammals, there are 11 major organ systems: **integumentary system, respiratory system, cardiovascular system, endocrine system, nervous system, immune system, digestive system, excretory system, muscular system, skeletal system,** and **reproductive system.**

Tissues are groups of cells that work together to perform a specific function. Tissues are divided into broad categories based on their function:
- **Epithelial** – Tissue in which cells are joined together tightly. *Skin* tissue is an example.
- **Connective** – Connective tissue may be dense, loose, or fatty. It protects and binds body parts. Connective tissues include *bone tissue, cartilage, tendons, ligaments, fat, blood, and lymph.*
- **Cartilage** – Cushions and provides structural support for body parts. It has a jelly-like base and is fibrous.
- **Blood** – Blood transports oxygen to cells and removes wastes. It also carries hormones and defends against disease.
- **Bone** – Bone is a hard tissue that supports and protects softer tissues and organs. Its marrow produces red blood cells.
- **Muscle** – Muscle tissue helps support and move the body. The three types of muscle tissue are *smooth, cardiac, and skeletal.*
- **Nervous** – Nerve tissue is located in the *brain, spinal cord, and nerves.* Cells called neurons form a network through the body that control responses to changes in the external and internal environment. Some send signals to muscles and glands to trigger responses.

Medial means *nearer to the midline* of the body. In anatomical position, the little finger is medial to the thumb.

Lateral is the opposite of medial. It refers to structures *further away from the body's midline*, at the sides. In anatomical position, the thumb is lateral to the little finger.

Proximal refers to structures *closer to the center* of the body. The hip is proximal to the knee.

Distal refers to structures *further away from the center* of the body. The knee is distal to the hip.

Anterior refers to structures in *front*.

Posterior refers to structures *behind*.

The **transverse (or horizontal) plane** divides the patient's body into imaginary upper (*superior*) and lower (*inferior* or *caudal*) halves.

The **sagittal plane** divides the body, or any body part, vertically into right and left sections. The sagittal plane runs parallel to the midline of the body.

The **coronal (or frontal) plane** divides the body, or any body structure, vertically into front and back (*anterior* and *posterior*) sections. The coronal plane runs vertically through the body at right angles to the midline.

Define the terms cephalad, caudad, superior, and inferior.

Explain the components of the upper and lower respiratory system.

Describe the main functions of the respiratory system.

Explain the function of the diaphragm during the breathing process.

List the parts of the circulatory system and discuss their purpose.

Describe and discuss blood.

The respiratory system can be divided into the upper and lower respiratory system. The **upper respiratory system** includes the nose, nasal cavity, mouth, pharynx, and larynx. The **lower respiratory system** includes the trachea, lungs, and bronchial tree. Alternatively, the components of the respiratory system can be categorized as part of the airway, the lungs, or the respiratory muscles. The **airway** includes the nose, nasal cavity, mouth, pharynx, (throat), larynx (voice box), trachea (windpipe), bronchi, and bronchial network. The airway is lined with **cilia** that trap microbes and debris and sweep them back toward the mouth. The **lungs** are structures that house the **bronchi** and bronchial network, which extend into the lungs and terminate in millions of **alveoli** (air sacs). The walls of the alveoli are only one cell thick, allowing for the exchange of gases with the blood capillaries that surround them. The right lung has three lobes. The left lung only has two lobes, leaving room for the heart on the left side of the body. The lungs are surrounded by a **pleural membrane**, which reduces friction between surfaces when breathing. The respiratory muscles include the **diaphragm** and the **intercostal muscles**. The diaphragm is a dome-shaped muscle that separates the thoracic and abdominal cavities. The intercostal muscles are located between the ribs.

Cephalad and **cephalic** are adverbs meaning towards the *head*. **Cranial** is the adjective, meaning of the *skull*.

Caudad is an adverb meaning towards the *tail* or posterior. **Caudal** is the adjective, meaning of the *hindquarters*.

Superior means *above*, or closer to the head.

Inferior means *below*, or closer to the feet.

During the breathing process, the **diaphragm** and the **intercostal muscles** contract to expand the lungs.

During **inspiration** or inhalation, the diaphragm contracts and moves down, increasing the size of the chest cavity. The intercostal muscles contract and the ribs expand, increasing the size of the **chest cavity**. As the volume of the chest cavity increases, the pressure inside the chest cavity decreases. Because the outside air is under a greater amount of pressure than the air inside the lungs, air rushes into the lungs.

When the diaphragm and intercostal muscles relax, the size of the chest cavity decreases, forcing air out of the lungs (**expiration** or exhalation). The breathing process is controlled by the portion of the brain stem called the **medulla oblongata**. The medulla oblongata monitors the level of carbon dioxide in the blood and signals the breathing rate to increase when these levels are too high.

The main function of the respiratory system is to supply the body with **oxygen** and rid the body of **carbon dioxide**. This exchange of gases occurs in millions of tiny **alveoli**, which are surrounded by blood capillaries.

The respiratory system also filters air. Air is warmed, moistened, and filtered as it passes through the nasal passages before it reaches the lungs.

The respiratory system is responsible for speech. As air passes through the throat, it moves through the **larynx** (voice box), which vibrates and produces sound, before it enters the **trachea** (windpipe). The respiratory system is vital in cough production. Foreign particles entering the nasal passages or airways are expelled from the body by the respiratory system.

The respiratory system functions in the sense of smell. **Chemoreceptors** that are located in the nasal cavity respond to airborne chemicals. The respiratory system also helps the body maintain acid-base **homeostasis**. Hyperventilation can increase blood pH during **acidosis** (low pH). Slowing breathing during **alkalosis** (high pH) helps to lower blood pH.

Blood helps maintain a healthy internal environment in animals by *carrying raw materials to cells* and *removing waste products*. It helps stabilize internal pH and hosts various kinds of infection fighters.

An adult human has about five quarts of blood. Blood is composed of **red and white blood cells, platelets**, and **plasma**. Plasma constitutes over half of the blood volume. It is mostly water and serves as a solvent. Plasma contains plasma proteins, ions, glucose, amino acids, hormones, and dissolved gases.

Red blood cells transport **oxygen** to cells. Red blood cells form in the bone marrow and can live for about four months. These cells are constantly being replaced by fresh ones, keeping the total number relatively stable.

White blood cells defend the body against **infection** and remove various wastes. The types of white blood cells include lymphocytes, neutrophils, monocytes, eosinophils, and basophils. **Platelets** are fragments of stem cells and serve an important function in *blood clotting*.

The **circulatory system** is responsible for the internal transport of substances to and from the cells. The circulatory system usually consists of the following three parts:

- **Blood** – Blood is composed of water, solutes, and other elements in a fluid connective tissue.
- **Blood Vessels** – Tubules of different sizes that transport blood.
- **Heart** – The heart is a muscular pump providing the pressure necessary to keep blood flowing.

Circulatory systems can be either **open** or **closed**. Most animals have closed systems, where the *heart and blood vessels are continually connected*. As the blood moves through the system from larger tubules through smaller ones, the rate slows down. The flow of blood in the **capillary beds**, the smallest tubules, is quite slow.
A supplementary system, the **lymph vascular system**, cleans up excess fluids and proteins and returns them to the circulatory system.

Describe the human heart and discuss how it works.

Visit *mometrix.com/academy* for related videos.
Enter video codes: 569724 and 783139

Describe the cardiac cycle.

Describe the three basic types of circulation including portal circulation and renal circulation as components of systemic circulation.

Define blood pressure and discuss its function.

Describe the lymphatic system and discuss its major functions.

Describe the anatomy of the spleen.

The cardiac cycle consists of **diastole** and **systole** phases, which can be further divided into the first and second phases to describe the events of the right and left sides of the heart. However, these events are simultaneously occurring. During the first diastole phase, blood flows through the **superior** and **inferior venae cavae**. Because the heart is relaxed, blood flows passively from the atrium through the open **atrioventricular valve** (tricuspid valve) to the right ventricle. The **sinoatrial (SA) node**, the cardiac pacemaker located in the wall of the right atrium, generates electrical signals, which are carried by the **Purkinje fibers** to the rest of the atrium, stimulating it to contract and fill the right ventricle with blood. The impulse from the SA node is transmitted to the ventricle through the atrioventricular (AV) node, signaling the right ventricle to contract and initiating the first systole phase. The tricuspid valve closes, and the **pulmonary semilunar valve** opens. Blood is pumped out the **pulmonary arteries** to the lungs. Blood returning from the lungs fills the left atrium as part of the second diastole phase. The SA node triggers the **mitral valve** to open, and blood fills the left ventricle. During the second systole phase, the mitral valve closes and the **aortic semilunar valve** opens. The left ventricle contracts, and blood is pumped out of the aorta to the rest of the body.

The heart is a muscular pump made of **cardiac muscle tissue**. It has four chambers; each half contains both an **atrium** and a **ventricle**, and the halves are separated by a valve, known as the AV valve. It is located between the ventricle and the artery leading away from the heart. Valves keep blood moving in a single direction and prevent any backwash into the chambers.

The heart has its own circulatory system with its own **coronary arteries**.

The heart functions by contracting and relaxing. **Atrial contraction** fills the ventricles and **ventricular contraction** empties them, forcing circulation. This sequence is called the **cardiac cycle**.

Cardiac muscles are attached to each other and signals for contractions spread rapidly. A complex electrical system controls the heartbeat as cardiac muscle cells produce and conduct electric signals. These muscles are said to be **self-exciting**, needing no external stimuli.

Blood pressure is the fluid pressure generated by the cardiac cycle. **Arterial blood pressure** functions by transporting oxygen-poor blood into the lungs and oxygen-rich blood to the body tissues. **Arteries** branch into smaller arterioles which contract and expand based on signals from the body. **Arterioles** are where adjustments are made in blood delivery to specific areas based on complex communication from body systems.

Capillary beds are diffusion sites for exchanges between blood and interstitial fluid. A capillary has the thinnest wall of any blood vessel, consisting of a single layer of **endothelial cells**.

Capillaries merge into venules, which in turn merge with larger diameter tubules called **veins**. Veins transport blood from body tissues *back to the heart*. Valves inside the veins facilitate this transport. The walls of veins are thin and contain smooth muscle and also function as blood volume reserves.

The **circulatory system** includes coronary circulation, pulmonary circulation, and systemic circulation. **Coronary circulation** is the flow of blood to the heart tissue. Blood enters the **coronary arteries**, which branch off the aorta, supplying major arteries, which enter the heart with oxygenated blood. The deoxygenated blood returns to the right atrium through the **cardiac veins**, which empty into the **coronary sinus**. **Pulmonary circulation** is the flow of blood between the heart and the lungs. Deoxygenated blood flows from the right ventricle to the lungs through **pulmonary arteries**. Oxygenated blood flows back to the left atrium through the **pulmonary veins**. **Systemic circulation** is the flow of blood to the entire body with the exception of coronary circulation and pulmonary circulation. Blood exits the left ventricle through the aorta, which branches into the *carotid arteries, subclavian arteries, common iliac arteries, and the renal artery*. Blood returns to the heart through the *jugular veins, subclavian veins, common iliac veins, and renal veins*, which empty into the **superior** and **inferior venae cavae**. Included in systemic circulation is **portal circulation**, which is the flow of blood from the digestive system to the liver and then to the heart, and **renal circulation**, which is the flow of blood between the heart and the kidneys.

The spleen is in the upper left of the abdomen. It is located behind the stomach and immediately below the diaphragm. It is about the size of a thick paperback book and weighs just over half a pound. It is made up of **lymphoid tissue**. The blood vessels are connected to the spleen by **splenic sinuses** (modified capillaries). The following **peritoneal ligaments** support the spleen:

- The **gastrolienal ligament** connects the stomach to the spleen.
- The **lienorenal ligament** connects the kidney to the spleen.
- The middle section of the **phrenicocolic ligament** (connects the left colic flexure to the thoracic diaphragm).

The main functions of the spleen are to *filter unwanted materials* from the blood (including old red blood cells) and to help *fight infections*. Up to ten percent of the population has one or more accessory spleens that tend to form at the **hilum** of the original spleen.

The main function of the **lymphatic system** is to *return excess tissue fluid to the bloodstream*. This system consists of transport vessels and lymphoid organs. The lymph vascular system consists of **lymph capillaries, lymph vessels, and lymph ducts**. The major functions of the lymph vascular system are:

- The return of excess fluid to the blood.
- The return of protein from the capillaries.
- The transport of fats from the digestive tract.
- The disposal of debris and cellular waste.

Lymphoid organs include the lymph nodes, spleen, appendix, adenoids, thymus, tonsils, and small patches of tissue in the small intestine. **Lymph nodes** are located at intervals throughout the lymph vessel system. Each node contains **lymphocytes** and **plasma cells**. The **spleen** filters blood stores of red blood cells and macrophages. The **thymus** secretes hormones and is the major site of lymphocyte production.

Science – Human Anatomy and Physiology
© Mometrix Media - flashcardsecrets.com/teas
ATI TEAS Exam

Give an overview of the digestive system.

Science – Human Anatomy and Physiology
© Mometrix Media - flashcardsecrets.com/teas
ATI TEAS Exam

Describe the mouth and stomach. List the three main functions of the stomach. State the purposes of the mouth and stomach.

Science – Human Anatomy and Physiology
© Mometrix Media - flashcardsecrets.com/teas
ATI TEAS Exam

Describe the general anatomy of the liver.

Science – Human Anatomy and Physiology
© Mometrix Media - flashcardsecrets.com/teas
ATI TEAS Exam

Describe the major functions of the liver.

Science – Human Anatomy and Physiology
© Mometrix Media - flashcardsecrets.com/teas
ATI TEAS Exam

Discuss the purpose of the small intestine in digestion.

Science – Human Anatomy and Physiology
© Mometrix Media - flashcardsecrets.com/teas
ATI TEAS Exam

Describe the large intestine and discuss its purpose.

Digestion begins in the mouth with the chewing and mixing of nutrients with **saliva**. Only humans and other mammals actually chew their food. **Salivary glands** are stimulated and secrete saliva. Saliva contains **enzymes** that initiate the breakdown of starch in digestion. Once swallowed, the food moves down the **pharynx** into the **esophagus** en route to the stomach.

The **stomach** is a flexible, muscular sac. It has three main functions:
- Mixing and storing food
- Dissolving and degrading food via secretions
- Controlling passage of food into the small intestine

Protein digestion begins in the stomach. Stomach acidity helps break down the food and make nutrients available for absorption. Smooth muscle moves the food by **peristalsis**, contracting and relaxing to move nutrients along. Smooth muscle contractions move nutrients into the small intestine where the **absorption** process begins.

Most digestive systems function by the following means:
- **Movement** – Movement mixes and passes nutrients through the system and eliminates waste.
- **Secretion** – Enzymes, hormones, and other substances necessary for digestion are secreted into the digestive tract.
- **Digestion** – Includes the chemical breakdown of nutrients into smaller units that enter the internal environment.
- **Absorption** – The passage of nutrients through plasma membranes into the blood or lymph and then to the body.

The liver is responsible for performing many vital functions in the body including:
- Production of **bile**
- Production of certain **blood plasma proteins**
- Production of **cholesterol** (and certain proteins needed to carry fats)
- Storage of excess glucose in the form of **glycogen** (that can be converted back to glucose when needed)
- Regulation of **amino acids**
- Processing of **hemoglobin** (to store iron)
- Conversion of ammonia (that is poisonous to the body) to **urea** (a waste product excreted in urine)
- **Purification** of the blood (clears out drugs and other toxins)
- Regulation of **blood clotting**
- Controlling infections by boosting **immune factors** and removing bacteria.

The nutrients (and drugs) that pass through the liver are converted into forms that are appropriate for the body to use.

The liver is the largest solid organ of the body. It is also the largest gland. It weighs about three pounds and is located below the diaphragm on the right side of the chest. The liver is made up of four **lobes**. They are called the *right, left, quadrate, and caudate lobes*. The liver is secured to the diaphragm and abdominal walls by five **ligaments**. They are called the *falciform* (that forms a membrane-like barrier between the right and left lobes), *coronary, right triangular, left triangular, and round ligaments*.

The liver processes all of the blood that passes through the digestive system. Nutrient-rich blood is supplied to the liver via the **hepatic portal vein**. The **hepatic artery** supplies oxygen-rich blood. Blood leaves the liver through the **hepatic veins**. The liver's functional units are called **lobules** (made up of layers of liver cells). Blood enters the lobules through branches of the portal vein and hepatic artery. The blood then flows through small channels called **sinusoids**.

Also called the **colon**, the large intestine concentrates, mixes, and stores waste material. A little over a meter in length, the colon ascends on the right side of the abdominal cavity, cuts across transversely to the left side, then descends and attaches to the **rectum**, a short tube for waste disposal.

When the rectal wall is distended by waste material, the nervous system triggers an impulse in the body to expel the waste from the rectum. A muscle **sphincter** at the end of the **anus** is stimulated to facilitate the expelling of waste matter.

The speed at which waste moves through the colon is influenced by the volume of fiber and other undigested material present. Without adequate bulk in the diet, it takes longer to move waste along, sometimes with negative effects. Lack of bulk in the diet has been linked to a number of disorders.

In the digestive process, most nutrients are absorbed in the **small intestine**. Enzymes from the pancreas, liver, and stomach are transported to the small intestine to aid digestion. These enzymes act on *fats, carbohydrates, nucleic acids, and proteins*. **Bile** is a secretion of the liver and is particularly useful in breaking down fats. It is stored in the **gall bladder** between meals.

By the time food reaches the lining of the small intestine, it has been reduced to small molecules. The lining of the small intestine is covered with **villi**, tiny absorptive structures that greatly increase the surface area for interaction with **chime** (the semi-liquid mass of partially digested food). Epithelial cells at the surface of the villi, called **microvilli**, further increase the ability of the small intestine to serve as the *main absorption organ* of the digestive tract.

Describe the general anatomy of the pancreas.

Describe the exocrine functions of the pancreas.

Give an overview of the human nervous system.

Describe the three general functional types of neurons.

Describe the two primary components of the central nervous system.

Discuss the role of the cerebellum in memory.

The pancreas assists in the digestion of foods by secreting **enzymes** (to the small intestine) that help to break down many foods, especially fats and proteins.

The precursors to these enzymes (called **zymogens**) are produced by groups of exocrine cells (called **acini**). They are converted, through a chemical reaction in the gut, to the active enzymes (such as **pancreatic lipase** and **amylase**) once they enter the small intestine. The pancreas also secretes large amounts of **sodium bicarbonate** to neutralize the stomach acid that reaches the small intestine.

The **exocrine** functions of the pancreas are controlled by hormones released by the stomach and small intestine (duodenum) when food is present. The exocrine secretions of the pancreas flow into the main pancreatic duct (**Wirsung's duct**) and are delivered to the duodenum through the pancreatic duct.

The pancreas is six to ten inches long and located at the back of the abdomen behind the stomach. It is a long, tapered organ. The wider (right) side is called the **head** and the narrower (left) side is called the **tail**. The head lies near the **duodenum** (the first part of the small intestine) and the tail ends near the **spleen**. The body of the pancreas lies between the head and the tail. The pancreas is made up of exocrine and endocrine tissues. The **exocrine tissue** secretes digestive enzymes from a series of ducts that collectively form the main pancreatic duct (that runs the length of the pancreas). The **main pancreatic duct** connects to the common bile duct near the duodenum. The **endocrine tissue** secretes hormones (such as insulin) into the bloodstream. Blood is supplied to the pancreas from the *splenic artery, gastroduodenal artery, and the superior mesenteric artery*.

The three general functional types of neurons are the sensory neurons, motor neurons, and interneurons. **Sensory neurons** transmit signals to the **central nervous system** (CNS) from the sensory receptors associated with touch, pain, temperature, hearing, sight, smell, and taste. **Motor neurons** transmit signals from the CNS to the rest of the body such as by signaling muscles or glands to respond. **Interneurons** transmit signals between neurons; for example, interneurons receive transmitted signals between sensory neurons and motor neurons. In general, a neuron consists of three basic parts: the cell body, the axon, and many dendrites. The **dendrites** receive **impulses** from sensory receptors or interneurons and transmit them toward the cell body. The **cell body** (soma) contains the nucleus of the neuron. The **axon** transmits the impulses away from the cell body. The axon is insulated by **oligodendrocytes** and the **myelin sheath** with gaps known as the **nodes of Ranvier**. The axon terminates at the synapse.

The human nervous system senses, interprets, and issues commands as a response to conditions in the body's environment. This process is made possible by a very complex communication system organized as a grid of **neurons**.

Messages are sent across the plasma membrane of neurons through a process called **action potential**. These messages occur when a neuron is stimulated past a necessary threshold. These stimulations occur in a sequence from the stimulation point of one neuron to its contact with another neuron. At the point of contact, called a **chemical synapse**, a substance is released that stimulates or inhibits the action of the adjoining cell. This network fans out across the body and forms the framework for the nervous system. The direction the information flows depends on the specific organizations of nerve circuits and pathways.

The **cerebellum** plays a role in the processing and storing of *implicit memories*. Specifically, for those memories developed during classical conditioning learning techniques. The role of the cerebellum was discovered by exploring the memory of individuals with damaged cerebellums. These individuals were unable to develop stimulus responses when presented via a classical conditioning technique. Researchers found that this was also the case for automatic responses. For example, when these individuals were presented with a puff of air into their eyes, they did not blink, which would have been the naturally occurring and automatic response in an individual with no brain damage.

Spinal Cord
The spinal cord is encased in the bony structure of the **vertebrae**, which protects and supports it. Its nervous tissue functions mainly with respect to limb movement and internal organ activity. Major nerve tracts ascend and descend from the spinal cord to the brain.
Brain
The brain consists of the hindbrain, midbrain, and forebrain. The **hindbrain** includes the **medulla oblongata**, **cerebellum**, and **pons**. The **midbrain** integrates sensory signals and orchestrates responses to these signals. The **forebrain** includes the **cerebrum**, **thalamus**, and **hypothalamus**. The **cerebral cortex** is a thin layer of gray matter covering the cerebrum. The brain is divided into two hemispheres, with each responsible for multiple functions. The brain is divided into four main **lobes**, the frontal lobe, the parietal lobe, the occipital lobe, and the temporal lobes. The **frontal lobe** located in the front of the brain is responsible for a short term and working *memory and information processing* as well as *decision-making, planning, and judgment*. The **parietal lobe** is located slightly toward the back of the brain and the top of the head and is responsible for *sensory input* as well as *spatial positioning of the body*. The **occipital lobe** is located at the back of the head just above the brain stem. This lobe is responsible for *visual input, processing, and output*; specifically nerves from the eyes enter directly into this lobe. Finally, the **temporal lobes** are located at the left and right sides of the brain. These lobes are responsible for all *auditory input, processing, and output*.

Science – Human Anatomy and Physiology
© Mometrix Media - flashcardsecrets.com/teas
ATI TEAS Exam

Describe the three parts of the brain stem. Briefly outline the peripheral nervous system.

Science – Human Anatomy and Physiology
© Mometrix Media - flashcardsecrets.com/teas
ATI TEAS Exam

Describe the autonomic nervous system and its role in homeostasis.

Visit *mometrix.com/academy* for a related video.
Enter video code: 708428

Science – Human Anatomy and Physiology
© Mometrix Media - flashcardsecrets.com/teas
ATI TEAS Exam

Describe the somatic nervous system and the reflex arc.

Science – Human Anatomy and Physiology
© Mometrix Media - flashcardsecrets.com/teas
ATI TEAS Exam

Describe the muscular system and list the three common properties of muscles.

Science – Human Anatomy and Physiology
© Mometrix Media - flashcardsecrets.com/teas
ATI TEAS Exam

Describe the three types of muscular tissue in the human body.

Science – Human Anatomy and Physiology
© Mometrix Media - flashcardsecrets.com/teas
ATI TEAS Exam

Describe the muscle fibers within skeletal muscles.

The autonomic nervous system (**ANS**) maintains **homeostasis** within the body. In general, the ANS controls the functions of the *internal organs, blood vessels, smooth muscle tissues, and glands*. This is accomplished through the direction of the **hypothalamus**, which is located above the midbrain. The hypothalamus controls the ANS through the brain stem. With this direction from the hypothalamus, the ANS helps maintain a stable body environment (homeostasis) by regulating numerous factors including heart rate, breathing rate, body temperature, and blood pH.

The ANS consists of two divisions: the sympathetic nervous system and the parasympathetic nervous system. The **sympathetic nervous system** controls the body's reaction to extreme, stressful, and emergency situations. For example, the sympathetic nervous system increases the heart rate, signals the adrenal glands to secrete adrenaline, triggers the dilation of the pupils, and slows digestion. The **parasympathetic nervous system** counteracts the effects of the sympathetic nervous system. For example, the parasympathetic nervous system decreases heart rate, signals the adrenal glands to stop secreting adrenaline, constricts the pupils, and returns the digestion process to normal.

The posterior area of the brain that is connected to the spinal cord is known as the **brain stem**. The **midbrain**, the **pons**, and the **medulla oblongata** are the three parts of the brain stem. Information from the body is sent to the brain through the brain stem, and information from the brain is sent to the body through the brain stem. The brain stem is an important part of *respiratory, digestive, and circulatory functions*.

The **midbrain** lies above the pons and the medulla oblongata. The parts of the midbrain include the **tectum**, the **tegmentum**, and the **ventral tegmentum**. The midbrain is an important part of *vision and hearing*. The **pons** comes between the midbrain and the medulla oblongata. Information is sent across the pons from the cerebrum to the medulla and the cerebellum. The **medulla oblongata** (or medulla) is beneath the midbrain and the pons. The medulla oblongata is the piece of the brain stem that connects the spinal cord to the brain. So, it has an important role with the autonomic nervous system in the *circulatory and respiratory system*.

The **peripheral nervous system** consists of the nerves and ganglia throughout the body and includes **sympathetic nerves** that trigger the "fight or flight" response, and the **parasympathetic nerves** which control basic body function.

There are three types of muscle tissue: **skeletal**, **cardiac**, and **smooth**. There are over 600 muscles in the human body. All muscles have these three properties in common:

- **Excitability** – All muscle tissues have an *electric gradient* which can reverse when stimulated.
- **Contraction** – All muscle tissues have the ability to contract, or *shorten*.
- **Elongate** – All muscle tissues share the capacity to elongate, or *relax*.

The somatic nervous system (**SNS**) controls the five senses and the voluntary movement of skeletal muscle. So, this system has all of the neurons that are connected to sense organs. Efferent (motor) and afferent (sensory) nerves help the somatic nervous system operate the senses and the movement of skeletal muscle. **Efferent nerves** bring signals from the central nervous system to the sensory organs and the muscles. **Afferent nerves** bring signals from the sensory organs and the muscles to the central nervous system. The somatic nervous system also performs involuntary movements which are known as reflex arcs.

A **reflex**, the simplest act of the nervous system, is an automatic response without any conscious thought to a stimulus via the reflex arc. The **reflex arc** is the simplest nerve pathway, which bypasses the brain and is controlled by the spinal cord. For example, in the classic knee-jerk response (patellar tendon reflex), the stimulus is the reflex hammer hitting the tendon, and the response is the muscle contracting, which jerks the foot upward. The stimulus is detected by sensory receptors, and a message is sent along a **sensory** (afferent) neuron to one or more **interneurons** in the spinal cord. The interneuron(s) transmit this message to a **motor** (efferent) neuron, which carries the message to the correct **effector** (muscle).

Skeletal muscles consist of numerous muscle fibers. Each muscle fiber contains a bundle of **myofibrils**, which are composed of multiple repeating contractile units called **sarcomeres**.

Myofibrils contain two protein **microfilaments**: a thick filament and a thin filament. The thick filament is composed of the protein **myosin**. The thin filament is composed of the protein **actin**. The dark bands (**striations**) in skeletal muscles are formed when thick and thin filaments overlap. Light bands occur where the thin filament is overlapped. Skeletal muscle attraction occurs when the thin filaments slide over the thick filaments, shortening the sarcomere.

When an **action potential** (electrical signal) reaches a muscle fiber, **calcium ions** are released. According to the sliding filament model of muscle contraction, these calcium ions bind to the myosin and actin, which assists in the binding of the **myosin heads** of the thick filaments to the **actin molecules** of the thin filaments. **Adenosine triphosphate** released from glucose provides the energy necessary for the contraction.

Skeletal muscles are *voluntary* muscles that work in pairs to move various parts of the skeleton. Skeletal muscles are composed of **muscle fibers** (cells) that are bound together in parallel **bundles**. Skeletal muscles are also known as **striated muscle** due to their striped appearance under a microscope.

Smooth muscle tissues are *involuntary* muscles that are found in the walls of internal organs such as the stomach, intestines, and blood vessels. Smooth muscle tissues or **visceral tissue** is nonstriated. Smooth muscle cells are shorter and wider than skeletal muscle fibers. Smooth muscle tissue is also found in sphincters or valves that control various openings throughout the body.

Cardiac muscle tissue is *involuntary* muscle that is found only in the heart. Like skeletal muscle cells, cardiac muscle cells are also striated.

Only skeletal muscle interacts with the skeleton to move the body. When they contract, the muscles transmit **force** to the attached bones. Working together, the muscles and bones act as a system of levers which move around the joints. A small contraction of a muscle can produce a large movement. A limb can be extended and rotated around a joint due to the way the muscles are arranged.

Describe the anatomy and function of the male reproductive system.

Describe the anatomy and functions of the female reproductive system.

Explain the integumentary system and its function.

Explain the layers of skin.

Describe temperature homeostasis and thermoregulation with the skin.

Describe sebaceous glands and sweat glands.

The functions of the female reproductive system are to produce **ova** (oocytes, or egg cells), transfer the ova to the **fallopian tubes** for fertilization, receive the sperm from the male, and to provide a protective, nourishing environment for the developing **embryo**.

The external portion of the female reproductive system includes the labia majora, labia minora, Bartholin's glands and clitoris. The **labia majora** and the **labia minora** enclose and protect the vagina. The **Bartholin's glands** secrete a lubricating fluid. The **clitoris** contains erectile tissue and nerve endings for sensual pleasure.

The internal portion of the female reproductive system includes the ovaries, fallopian tubes, uterus, and vagina. The **ovaries**, which are the female gonads, produce the ova and secrete **estrogen** and **progesterone**. The **fallopian tubes** carry the mature egg toward the uterus. Fertilization typically occurs in the fallopian tubes. If fertilized, the egg travels to the **uterus**, where it implants in the uterine wall. The uterus protects and nourishes the developing embryo until birth. The **vagina** is a muscular tube that extends from the **cervix** of the uterus to the outside of the body. The vagina receives the semen and sperm during sexual intercourse and provides a birth canal when needed.

The functions of the male reproductive system are to produce, maintain, and transfer **sperm** and **semen** into the female reproductive tract and to produce and secrete **male hormones**.

The external structure includes the penis, scrotum, and testes. The **penis**, which contains the **urethra**, can fill with blood and become erect, enabling the deposition of semen and sperm into the female reproductive tract during sexual intercourse. The **scrotum** is a sac of skin and smooth muscle that houses the testes and keeps the testes at the proper temperature for **spermatogenesis**. The **testes**, or testicles, are the male gonads, which produce sperm and testosterone.

The internal structure includes the epididymis, vas deferens, ejaculatory ducts, urethra, seminal vesicles, prostate gland, and bulbourethral glands. The **epididymis** stores the sperm as it matures. Mature sperm moves from the epididymis through the **vas deferens** to the **ejaculatory duct**. The **seminal vesicles** secrete alkaline fluids with proteins and mucus into the ejaculatory duct, also. The **prostate gland** secretes a milky white fluid with proteins and enzymes as part of the semen. The **bulbourethral**, or Cowper's, glands secrete a fluid into the urethra to neutralize the acidity in the urethra.

Additionally, the hormones associated with the male reproductive system include **follicle-stimulating hormone**, which stimulates spermatogenesis; **luteinizing hormone**, which stimulates testosterone production; and **testosterone**, which is responsible for the male sex characteristics.

The layers of the skin from the surface of the skin inward are the epidermis and dermis. The subcutaneous layer lying below the dermis is also part of the integumentary system. The **epidermis** is the most superficial layer of the skin. The epidermis, which consists entirely of **epithelial cells**, does not contain any blood vessels. The deepest portion of the epidermis is the **stratum basale**, which is a single layer of cells that continually undergo division. As more and more cells are produced, older cells are pushed toward the surface. Most epidermal cells are keratinized. **Keratin** is a waxy protein that helps to waterproof the skin. As the cells die, they are sloughed off. The **dermis** lies directly beneath the epidermis. The dermis consists mostly of connective tissue. The dermis contains blood vessels, sensory receptors, hair follicles, sebaceous glands, and sweat glands. The dermis also contains **elastin** and **collagen fibers**. The **subcutaneous layer** or **hypodermis** is actually not a layer of the skin. The subcutaneous layer consists of connective tissue, which binds the skin to the underlying muscles. Fat deposits in the subcutaneous layer help to cushion and insulate the body.

The integumentary system, which consists of the skin including the sebaceous glands, sweat glands, hair, and nails, serves a variety of functions associated with protection, secretion, and communication. In the functions associated with protection, the integumentary system protects the body from **pathogens** including bacteria, viruses, and various chemicals. In the functions associated with secretion, **sebaceous glands** secrete **sebum** (oil) that waterproofs the skin, and **sweat glands** are associated with the body's homeostatic relationship of **thermoregulation**. Sweat glands also serve as excretory organs and help rid the body of metabolic wastes. In the functions associated with communication, **sensory receptors** distributed throughout the skin send information to the brain regarding pain, touch, pressure, and temperature. In addition to protection, secretion, and communication, the skin manufactures **vitamin D** and can absorb certain chemicals such as specific medications.

Sebaceous glands and sweat glands are exocrine glands found in the skin. **Exocrine glands** secrete substances into **ducts**. In this case, the secretions are through the ducts to the surface of the skin.

Sebaceous glands are **holocrine glands**, which secrete sebum. **Sebum** is an oily mixture of lipids and proteins. Sebaceous glands are connected to hair follicles and secrete sebum through the hair pore. Sebum inhibits water loss from the skin and protects against bacterial and fungal infections.

Sweat glands are either eccrine glands or apocrine glands. **Eccrine glands** are not connected to hair follicles. They are activated by elevated body temperature. Eccrine glands are located throughout the body and can be found on the forehead, neck, and back. Eccrine glands secrete a salty solution of electrolytes and water containing sodium chloride, potassium, bicarbonate, glucose, and antimicrobial peptides.

Eccrine glands are activated as part of the body's thermoregulation. **Apocrine glands** secrete an oily solution containing fatty acids, triglycerides, and proteins. Apocrine glands are located in the armpits, groin, palms, and soles of the feet. Apocrine glands secrete this oily sweat when a person experiences stress or anxiety. Bacteria feed on apocrine sweat and expel aromatic fatty acids, producing body odor.

The skin is involved in **temperature homeostasis** or thermoregulation through the activation of the sweat glands. By **thermoregulation**, the body maintains a stable body temperature as one component of a stable internal environment. The temperature of the body is controlled by a negative feedback system consisting of a receptor, control center, and effector. The **receptors** are sensory cells located in the dermis of the skin. The **control center** is the **hypothalamus**, which is located in the brain. The **effectors** include the *sweat glands, blood vessels, and muscles* (shivering). The evaporation of sweat across the surface of the skin cools the body to maintain its tolerance range. **Vasodilation** of the blood vessels near the surface of the skin also releases heat into the environment to lower body temperature. Shivering is associated with the muscular system.

Give an overview of the endocrine system.

List the eight major endocrine glands and their functions.

Describe the endocrine functions of the pancreas.

Describe the location and function of the thyroid gland and parathyroid glands.

Briefly outline the renal/urinary system.

Describe the general structure of the kidneys and explain how they filter the blood.

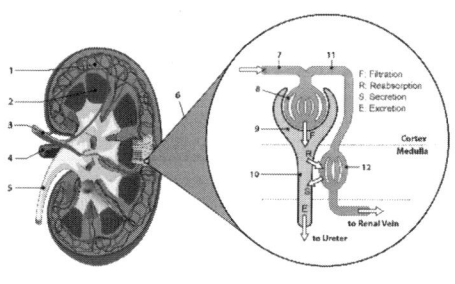

The eight major endocrine glands and their functions are:

- **Adrenal cortex** – Monitors blood sugar level; helps in lipid and protein metabolism.
- **Adrenal medulla** – Controls cardiac function; raises blood sugar and controls the size of blood vessels.
- **Thyroid gland** – Helps regulate metabolism and functions in growth and development.
- **Parathyroid** – Regulates calcium levels in the blood.
- **Pancreas islets** – Raises and lowers blood sugar; active in carbohydrate metabolism.
- **Thymus gland** – Plays a role in immune responses.
- **Pineal gland** – Has an influence on daily biorhythms and sexual activity.
- **Pituitary gland** – Plays an important role in growth and development.

Endocrine glands are intimately involved in a myriad of reactions, functions, and secretions that are crucial to the well-being of the body.

The endocrine system is responsible for secreting the **hormones** and other molecules that help regulate the entire body in both the short and the long term. There is a close working relationship between the endocrine system and the nervous system. The **hypothalamus** and the **pituitary gland** coordinate to serve as a **neuroendocrine control center**.

Hormone secretion is triggered by a variety of signals, including hormonal signs, chemical reactions, and environmental cues. Only cells with particular **receptors** can benefit from hormonal influence. This is the "key in the lock" model for hormonal action. **Steroid hormones** trigger gene activation and protein synthesis in some target cells. **Protein hormones** change the activity of existing enzymes in target cells. Hormones such as **insulin** work quickly when the body signals an urgent need. Slower acting hormones afford longer, gradual, and sometimes permanent changes in the body.

The thyroid and parathyroid glands are located in the neck just below the larynx. The parathyroid glands are four small glands that are embedded on the posterior side of the thyroid gland.

The basic function of the **thyroid gland** is to regulate metabolism. The thyroid gland secretes the hormones thyroxine, triiodothyronine, and calcitonin. **Thyroxine** and **triiodothyronine** increase metabolism, and **calcitonin** decreases blood calcium by storing calcium in bone tissue.

The **hypothalamus** directs the pituitary gland to secrete **thyroid-stimulating hormone** (TSH), which stimulates the thyroid gland to release these hormones as needed via a negative-feedback mechanism. The **parathyroid glands** secrete **parathyroid hormone**, which can increase blood calcium by moving calcium from the bone to the blood.

Located amongst the groupings of **exocrine cells** (acini) are groups of **endocrine cells** (called islets of Langerhans). The **islets of Langerhans** are primarily made up of insulin-producing **beta cells** (fifty to eighty percent of the total) and glucagon-releasing **alpha cells**.

The major hormones produced by the pancreas are insulin and glucagon. The body uses **insulin** to control carbohydrate metabolism by *lowering* the amount of sugar (**glucose**) in the blood. Insulin also affects fat **metabolism** and can change the liver's ability to release stored fat. The body also uses **glucagon** to control carbohydrate metabolism. Glucagon has the opposite effect of insulin in that the body uses it to *increase* blood sugar (glucose) levels. The levels of insulin and glucagon are balanced to maintain the optimum level of blood sugar (glucose) throughout the day.

The kidneys are bean-shaped structures that are located at the back of the abdominal cavity just under the diaphragm. Each **kidney** consists of three layers: the renal cortex (outer layer), renal medulla (inner layer), and renal pelvis (innermost portion).

The **renal cortex** is composed of approximately one million **nephrons**, which are the tiny, individual filters of the kidneys. Each nephron contains a cluster of capillaries called a **glomerulus** surrounded by the cup-shaped **Bowman's capsule**, which leads to a tubule.

The kidneys receive blood from the **renal arteries**, which branch off the aorta. In general, the kidneys filter the blood, reabsorb needed materials, and secrete wastes and excess water in the urine. More specifically, blood flows from the renal arteries into **arterioles** into the glomerulus, where it is filtered. The **glomerular filtrate** enters the **proximal convoluted tubule** where water, glucose, ions, and other organic molecules are reabsorbed back into the bloodstream.

Additional substances such as urea and drugs are removed from the blood in the **distal convoluted tubule**. Also, the pH of the blood can be adjusted in the distal convoluted tubule by the secretion of **hydrogen ions**. Finally, the unabsorbed materials flow out from the collecting tubules located in the **renal medulla** to the **renal pelvis** as urine. Urine is drained from the kidneys through the **ureters** to the **urinary bladder**, where it is stored until expulsion from the body through the **urethra**.

The urinary system is capable of eliminating excess substances while preserving the substances needed by the body to function. The **urinary system** consists of the kidneys, urinary ducts, and bladder.

Discuss the function of the immune system.

List and describe general nonspecific defense responses of the immune system.

List and describe specific defense responses of the immune system.

Discuss the types and functions of lymph nodes.

Discuss antigens and their functions.

Discuss active and passive immunity.

The body's general immune defenses include:
- **Skin** – An intact epidermis and dermis form a formidable barrier against bacteria.
- **Ciliated Mucous Membranes** – Cilia sweep pathogens out of the respiratory tract.
- **Glandular Secretions** – Secretions from exocrine glands destroy bacteria.
- **Gastric Secretions** – Gastric acid destroys pathogens.
- **Normal Bacterial Populations** – Compete with pathogens in the gut and vagina.

In addition, **phagocytes** and inflammation responses mobilize white blood cells and chemical reactions to stop infection. These responses include localized redness, tissue repair, and fluid-seeping healing agents. Additionally, **plasma proteins** act as the complement system to repel bacteria and pathogens.

The immune system protects the body against invading **pathogens** including bacteria, viruses, fungi, and protists. The immune system includes the **lymphatic system** (lymph, lymph capillaries, lymph vessel, and lymph nodes) as well as the **red bone marrow** and numerous **leukocytes**, or white blood cells. Tissue fluid enters the **lymph capillaries**, which combine to form **lymph vessels**. Skeletal muscle contractions move the lymph one way through the lymphatic system to lymphatic ducts, which dump back into the venous blood supply into the **lymph nodes**, which are situated along the lymph vessels, and filter the lymph of pathogens and other matter. The lymph nodes are concentrated in the neck, armpits, and groin areas. Outside the lymphatic vessel system lies the **lymphatic tissue** including the tonsils, adenoids, thymus, spleen, and Peyer's patches. The **tonsils**, located in the pharynx, protect against pathogens entering the body through the mouth and throat. The **thymus** serves as a maturation chamber for the immature T cells that are formed in the bone marrow. The **spleen** cleans the blood of dead cells and pathogens. **Peyer's patches**, which are located in the small intestine, protect the digestive system from pathogens.

Leukocytes, or white blood cells, are produced in the red bone marrow. Leukocytes can be classified as **monocytes** (macrophages and dendritic cells), **granulocytes** (neutrophils, basophils, and eosinophils), **T lymphocytes**, **B lymphocytes**, or **natural killer cells**.

Macrophages found traveling in the lymph or fixed in lymphatic tissue are the largest, long-living phagocytes that engulf and destroy pathogens. **Dendritic cells** present antigens (foreign particles) to T cells. **Neutrophils** are short-living phagocytes that respond quickly to invaders. **Basophils** alert the body of invasion. **Eosinophils** are large, long-living phagocytes that defend against multicellular invaders.

T lymphocytes or T cells include helper T cells, killer T cells, suppressor T cells, and memory T cells. **Helper T cells** help the body fight infections by producing antibodies and other chemicals. **Killer T cells** destroy cells that are infected with a virus or pathogen and tumor cells. **Suppressor T cells** stop or "suppress" the other T cells when the battle is over. **Memory T cells** remain in the blood on alert in case the invader attacks again. **B lymphocytes**, or B cells, produce antibodies.

Three types of white blood cells form the foundation of the body's immune system:
- **Macrophages** – Phagocytes that alert T cells to the presence of foreign substances.
- **T Lymphocytes** – These directly attack cells infected by viruses and bacteria.
- **B Lymphocytes** – These cells target specific bacteria for destruction.

Memory cells, **suppressor T cells**, and **helper T cells** also contribute to the body's defense. Immune responses can be **antibody-mediated** when the response is to an antigen, or **cell-mediated** when the response is to already infected cells. These responses are controlled and measured counterattacks that recede when the foreign agents are destroyed. Once an invader has attacked the body, if it returns it is immediately recognized and a secondary immune response occurs. This secondary response is rapid and powerful, much more so than the original response. These memory lymphocytes circulate throughout the body for years, alert to a possible new attack.

At birth, an **innate immune system** protects an individual from pathogens. When an individual encounters infection or has an immunization, the individual develops an **adaptive immunity** that reacts to pathogens. So, this adaptive immunity is acquired. Active and passive immunities can be acquired naturally or artificially.

A **naturally acquired active immunity** is natural because the individual is exposed and builds immunity to a pathogen *without an immunization*. An **artificially acquired active immunity** is artificial because the individual is exposed and builds immunity to a pathogen *by a vaccine*.

A **naturally acquired passive immunity** is natural because it happens *during pregnancy* as antibodies move from the mother's bloodstream to the bloodstream of the fetus. The antibodies can also be transferred from a mother's breast milk. During infancy, these antibodies provide temporary protection until childhood.

An **artificially acquired passive immunity** is an *immunization* that is given in recent outbreaks or emergency situations. This immunization provides quick and short-lived protection to disease by the use of antibodies that can come from another person or animal.

Antigens are substances that stimulate the **immune system**. Antigens are typically proteins on the surfaces of bacteria, viruses, and fungi.

Substances such as drugs, toxins, and foreign particles can also be antigens. The human body recognizes the antigens of its own cells, but it will attack cells or substances with unfamiliar antigens.

Specific **antibodies** are produced for each antigen that enters the body. In a typical immune response, when a pathogen or foreign substance enters the body, it is engulfed by a **macrophage**, which presents fragments of the antigen on its surface. A **helper T cell** joins the macrophage, and the killer (cytotoxic) T cells and B cells are activated. **Killer T cells** search out and destroy cells presenting the same antigens. **B cells** differentiate into plasma cells and memory cells.

Plasma cells produce antibodies specific to that pathogen or foreign substance. **Antibodies** bind to antigens on the surface of pathogens and mark them for destruction by other phagocytes. **Memory cells** remain in the blood stream to protect against future infections from the same pathogen.

Science – Human Anatomy and Physiology
© Mometrix Media - flashcardsecrets.com/teas
ATI TEAS Exam

Describe the skeletal system in the human body.

Science – Human Anatomy and Physiology
© Mometrix Media - flashcardsecrets.com/teas
ATI TEAS Exam

Discuss the components of the human skeleton.

Science – Human Anatomy and Physiology
© Mometrix Media - flashcardsecrets.com/teas
ATI TEAS Exam

Describe the function of the skeletal system.

Science – Human Anatomy and Physiology
© Mometrix Media - flashcardsecrets.com/teas
ATI TEAS Exam

Describe the role of the skeletal system.

Science – Human Anatomy and Physiology
© Mometrix Media - flashcardsecrets.com/teas
ATI TEAS Exam

Describe the components of the skeletal system.

Science – Human Anatomy and Physiology
© Mometrix Media - flashcardsecrets.com/teas
ATI TEAS Exam

Discuss the two types of connective bone tissue: compact and spongy.

The human skeletal system, which consists of 206 bones along with numerous tendons, ligaments, and cartilage, is divided into the axial skeleton and the appendicular skeleton. The **axial skeleton** consists of 80 bones and includes the vertebral column, rib cage, sternum, skull, and hyoid bone. The **vertebral column** consists of 33 vertebrae classified as cervical vertebrae, thoracic vertebrae, lumbar vertebrae, and sacral vertebrae. The **rib cage** includes 12 paired ribs, 10 pairs of true ribs and 2 pairs of floating ribs, and the **sternum**, which consists of the manubrium, corpus sterni, and xiphoid process. The **skull** includes the cranium and facial bones. The **ossicles** are bones in the middle ear. The **hyoid bone** provides an attachment point for the tongue muscles. The **axial skeleton** protects vital organs including the brain, heart, and lungs. The **appendicular skeleton** consists of 126 bones including the pectoral girdle, pelvic girdle, and appendages. The **pectoral girdle** consists of the scapulae (shoulders) and clavicles (collarbones). The **pelvic girdle** consists of two pelvic (hip) bones, which attach to the sacrum. The **upper appendages** (arms) include the humerus, radius, ulna, carpals, metacarpals, and phalanges. The **lower appendages** (legs) include the femur, patella, fibula, tibia, tarsals, metatarsals, and phalanges.

The skeletal structure in humans contains both **bones** and **cartilage**. Over 200 bones in the human body can be divided into two parts:

- **Axial skeleton** – Includes the skull, sternum, ribs, and vertebral column (the spine).
- **Appendicular skeleton** – Includes the bones of the arms, feet, hands, legs, hips, and shoulders.

The skeletal system has an important role in the following body functions:
- **Movement** – The action of skeletal muscles on bones moves the body.
- **Mineral Storage** – Bones serve as storage facilities for essential mineral ions.
- **Support** – Bones act as a framework and support system for the organs.
- **Protection** – Bones surround and protect key organs in the body.
- **Blood Cell Formation** – Red blood cells are produced in the marrow of certain bones.

The skeletal system serves many functions including providing structural support, providing movement, providing protection, producing blood cells, and storing substances such as fat and minerals. The skeletal system provides the body with structure and support for the muscles and organs. The axial skeleton transfers the weight from the upper body to the lower appendages. The skeletal system provides movement with **joints** and the muscular system. Bones provide attachment points for muscles. Joints including **hinge joints**, **ball-and-socket joints**, **pivot joints**, **ellipsoid joints**, **gliding joints**, and **saddle joints**. Each muscle is attached to two bones: the origin and the insertion. The **origin** remains immobile, and the **insertion** is the bone that moves as the muscle contracts and relaxes. The skeletal system serves to protect the body. The **cranium** protects the brain. The **vertebrae** protect the spinal cord. The **rib cage** protects the heart and lungs. The **pelvis** protects the reproductive organs. The **red marrow** manufactures red and white blood cells. All bone marrow is red at birth, but adults have approximately one-half red bone marrow and one-half yellow bone marrow. **Yellow bone marrow** stores fat. Also, the skeletal system provides a reservoir to store the minerals **calcium** and **phosphorus**.

Compact, or **cortical**, bone, which consists of tightly packed cells, is strong, dense, and rigid. Running vertically throughout compact bone are the **Haversian canals**, which are surrounded by concentric circles of bone tissue called **lamellae**. The spaces between the lamellae are called the **lacunae**. These lamellae and canals along with their associated arteries, veins, lymph vessels, and nerve endings are referred to collectively as the **Haversian system**.
The Haversian system provides a reservoir for calcium and phosphorus for the blood. Also, bones have a thin outside layer of compact bone, which gives them their characteristic smooth, white appearance.

Spongy, or **cancellous**, bone consists of **trabeculae**, which are a network of girders with open spaces filled with red bone marrow. Compared to compact bone, spongy bone is lightweight and porous, which helps reduce the bone's overall weight. The red marrow manufactures red and white blood cells. In long bones, the **diaphysis** consists of compact bone surrounding the marrow cavity and spongy bone containing red marrow in the **epiphyses**. Bones have varying amounts of compact bone and spongy bone depending on their classification.

Bones are classified as long, short, flat, or irregular. They are a connective tissue with a base of pulp containing **collagen** and living cells. Bone tissue is constantly regenerating itself as the mineral composition changes. This allows for special needs during growth periods and maintains calcium levels for the body. Bone regeneration can deteriorate in old age, particularly among women, leading to **osteoporosis**.

The flexible and curved **backbone** is supported by muscles and ligaments. **Intervertebral discs** are stacked one above another and provide cushioning for the backbone. Trauma or shock may cause these discs to **herniate** and cause pain. The sensitive **spinal cord** is enclosed in a cavity which is well protected by the bones of the vertebrae.

Joints are areas of contact adjacent to bones. **Synovial joints** are the most common, and are freely moveable. These may be found at the shoulders and knees. **Cartilaginous joints** fill the spaces between some bones and restrict movement. Examples of cartilaginous joints are those between vertebrae. **Fibrous joints** have fibrous tissue connecting bones and no cavity is present

Science – Life and Physical Sciences

Describe macromolecules and their function.

Science – Life and Physical Sciences

Describe carbohydrates and their functions.

Science – Life and Physical Sciences

Describe lipids and their functions.

Visit *mometrix.com/academy* for a related video.
Enter video code: 269746

Science – Life and Physical Sciences

Discuss proteins and their functions.

Visit *mometrix.com/academy* for a related video.
Enter video code: 903713

Science – Life and Physical Sciences

Give an overview of enzymes.

Science – Life and Physical Sciences

Describe nucleic acids and their functions.

Visit *mometrix.com/academy* for a related video.
Enter video code: 503931

Carbohydrates are the primary source of energy and are responsible for providing energy as they can be easily converted to **glucose**. It is the oxidation of carbohydrates that provides the cells with most of their energy. Glucose can be further broken down by respiration or fermentation by **glycolysis**. They are involved in the metabolic energy cycles of photosynthesis and respiration.

Structurally, carbohydrates usually take the form of some variation of CH_2O as they are made of carbon, hydrogen, and oxygen. Carbohydrates (**polysaccharides**) are broken down into sugars or glucose.

The simple sugars can be grouped into monosaccharides (glucose, fructose, and galactose) and disaccharides. These are both types of carbohydrates. Monosaccharides have one monomer of sugar and disaccharides have two. Monosaccharides (CH_2O) have one carbon for every water molecule.

A **monomer** is a small molecule. It is a single compound that forms chemical bonds with other monomers to make a polymer. A **polymer** is a compound of large molecules formed by repeating monomers. Carbohydrates, proteins, and nucleic acids are groups of macromolecules that are polymers.

Macromolecules are large and complex, and play an important role in cell structure and function. The four basic organic macromolecules produced by anabolic reactions are **carbohydrates** (polysaccharides), **nucleic acids**, **proteins**, and **lipids**. The four basic building blocks involved in catabolic reactions are **monosaccharides** (glucose), **amino acids**, **fatty acids** (glycerol), and **nucleotides**.

An **anabolic reaction** is one that builds larger and more complex molecules (macromolecules) from smaller ones. **Catabolic reactions** are the opposite. Larger molecules are broken down into smaller, simpler molecules. Catabolic reactions *release energy*, while anabolic ones *require energy*.

Endothermic reactions are chemical reactions that *absorb* heat and **exothermic reactions** are chemical reactions that *release* heat.

Proteins are macromolecules formed from amino acids. They are **polypeptides**, which consist of many (10 to 100) peptides linked together. The peptide connections are the result of condensation reactions. A **condensation reaction** results in a loss of water when two molecules are joined together. A **hydrolysis reaction** is the opposite of a condensation reaction. During hydrolysis, water is added. –H is added to one of the smaller molecules and OH is added to another molecule being formed. A **peptide** is a compound of two or more amino acids. **Amino acids** are formed by the partial hydrolysis of protein, which forms an **amide bond**. This partial hydrolysis involves an amine group and a carboxylic acid. In the carbon chain of amino acids, there is a **carboxylic acid group** (–COOH), an **amine group** (–NH_2), a **central carbon atom** between them with an attached hydrogen, and an attached **"R" group** (side chain), which is different for different amino acids. It is the "R" group that determines the properties of the protein.

Lipids are molecules that are soluble in nonpolar solvents, but are hydrophobic, meaning they do not bond well with water or mix well with water solutions. Lipids have numerous **C–H bonds**. In this way, they are similar to **hydrocarbons** (substances consisting only of carbon and hydrogen). The major roles of lipids include *energy storage and structural functions*. Examples of lipids include fats, phospholipids, steroids, and waxes. **Fats** (which are triglycerides) are made of long chains of fatty acids (three fatty acids bound to a glycerol). **Fatty acids** are chains with reduced carbon at one end and a carboxylic acid group at the other. An example is soap, which contains the sodium salts of free fatty acids. **Phospholipids** are lipids that have a phosphate group rather than a fatty acid. **Glycerides** are another type of lipid. Examples of glycerides are fat and oil. Glycerides are formed from fatty acids and glycerol (a type of alcohol).

Nucleic acids are macromolecules that are composed of **nucleotides**. Hydrolysis is a reaction in which water is broken down into **hydrogen cations** (H or H+) and **hydroxide anions** (OH or OH-). This is part of the process by which nucleic acids are broken down by enzymes to produce shorter strings of RNA and DNA (oligonucleotides). **Oligonucleotides** are broken down into smaller sugar nitrogenous units called **nucleosides**. These can be digested by cells since the sugar is divided from the nitrogenous base. This, in turn, leads to the formation of the five types of nitrogenous bases, sugars, and the preliminary substances involved in the synthesis of new RNA and DNA. DNA and RNA have a helix shape.

Macromolecular nucleic acid polymers, such as RNA and DNA, are formed from nucleotides, which are monomeric units joined by **phosphodiester bonds**. Cells require energy in the form of ATP to synthesize proteins from amino acids and replicate DNA. **Nitrogen fixation** is used to synthesize nucleotides for DNA and amino acids for proteins. Nitrogen fixation uses the enzyme nitrogenase in the reduction of dinitrogen gas (N_2) to ammonia (NH_3).

Nucleic acids store information and energy and are also important catalysts. It is the **RNA** that catalyzes the transfer of **DNA genetic information** into protein coded information. ATP is an RNA nucleotide. **Nucleotides** are used to form the nucleic acids. Nucleotides are made of a five-carbon sugar, such as ribose or deoxyribose, a nitrogenous base, and one or more phosphates. Nucleotides consisting of more than one phosphate can also store energy in their bonds.

Enzymes are proteins with strong **catalytic** power. They greatly accelerate the speed at which specific reactions approach equilibrium. Although enzymes do not start chemical reactions that would not eventually occur by themselves, they do make these reactions happen *faster and more often*. This acceleration can be substantial, sometimes making reactions happen a million times faster. Each type of enzyme deals with **reactants**, also called **substrates**. Each enzyme is highly selective, only interacting with substrates that are a match for it at an active site on the enzyme. This is the "key in the lock" analogy: a certain enzyme only fits with certain substrates. Even with a matching substrate, sometimes an enzyme must reshape itself to fit well with the substrate, forming a strong bond that aids in catalyzing a reaction before it returns to its original shape. An unusual quality of enzymes is that they are not permanently consumed in the reactions they speed up. They can be used again and again, providing a constant source of energy accelerants for cells. This allows for a tremendous increase in the number and rate of reactions in cells.

List some facts about DNA.

Visit *mometrix.com/academy* for a related video.
Enter video code: 639552

Discuss the structure of DNA.

Discuss purine bases and pyrimidine bases.

Define and discuss codons.

Discuss DNA replication.

Describe RNA and its three types.

DNA has a double helix shape, resembles a twisted ladder, and is compact. It consists of **nucleotides**. Nucleotides consist of a **five-carbon sugar** (pentose), a **phosphate group**, and a **nitrogenous base**. Two bases pair up to form the rungs of the ladder. The "side rails" or backbone consists of the covalently bonded sugar and phosphate. The bases are attached to each other with hydrogen bonds, which are easily dismantled so replication can occur. Each base is attached to a phosphate and to a sugar. There are four types of nitrogenous bases: **adenine** (A), **guanine** (G), **cytosine** (C), and **thymine** (T). There are about 3 billion bases in human DNA. The bases are mostly the same in everybody, but their order is different. It is the order of these bases that creates diversity in people. *Adenine (A) pairs with thymine (T)*, and *cytosine (C) pairs with guanine (G)*.

Chromosomes consist of **genes**, which are single units of genetic information. Genes are made up of deoxyribonucleic acid (DNA). DNA is a nucleic acid located in the cell nucleus. There is also DNA in the **mitochondria**. DNA replicates to pass on genetic information. The DNA in almost all cells is the same. It is also involved in the biosynthesis of proteins.

The model or structure of DNA is described as a **double helix**. A helix is a curve, and a double helix is two congruent curves connected by horizontal members. The model can be likened to a spiral staircase. It is right-handed. The British scientist Rosalind Elsie Franklin is credited with taking the x-ray diffraction image in 1952 that was used by Francis Crick and James Watson to formulate the double-helix model of DNA and speculate about its important role in carrying and transferring genetic information.

Codons are groups of three nucleotides on the messenger RNA, and can be visualized as three rungs of a ladder. A **codon** has the code for a single amino acid. There are 64 codons but 20 amino acids. More than one combination, or triplet, can be used to synthesize the necessary amino acids. For example, AAA (adenine-adenine-adenine) or AAG (adenine-adenine-guanine) can serve as codons for lysine. These groups of three occur in strings, and might be thought of as frames. For example, AAAUCUUCGU, if read in groups of three from the beginning, would be AAA, UCU, UCG, which are codons for lysine, serine, and serine, respectively. If the same sequence was read in groups of three starting from the second position, the groups would be AAU (asparagine), CUU (proline), and so on. The resulting amino acids would be completely different. For this reason, there are **start and stop codons** that indicate the beginning and ending of a sequence (or frame). **AUG** (methionine) is the start codon. **UAA**, **UGA**, and **UAG**, also known as ocher, opal, and amber, respectively, are stop codons.

The five bases in DNA and RNA can be categorized as either pyrimidine or purine according to their structure. The **pyrimidine bases** include *cytosine, thymine, and uracil*. They are six-sided and have a single ring shape. The **purine bases** are *adenine and guanine*, which consist of two attached rings. One ring has five sides and the other has six. When combined with a sugar, any of the five bases become **nucleosides**. Nucleosides formed from purine bases end in "osine" and those formed from pyrimidine bases end in "idine." **Adenosine** and **thymidine** are examples of nucleosides. Bases are the most basic components, followed by nucleosides, nucleotides, and then DNA or RNA.

RNA acts as a *helper* to DNA and carries out a number of other functions. Types of RNA include ribosomal RNA (rRNA), transfer RNA (tRNA), and messenger RNA (mRNA). Viruses can use RNA to carry their genetic material to DNA. **Ribosomal RNA** is not believed to have changed much over time. For this reason, it can be used to study relationships in organisms. **Messenger RNA** carries a copy of a strand of DNA and transports it from the nucleus to the cytoplasm. **Transcription** is the process in which RNA polymerase copies DNA into RNA. DNA unwinds itself and serves as a template while RNA is being assembled. The DNA molecules are copied to RNA. **Translation** is the process whereby ribosomes use transcribed RNA to put together the needed protein. **Transfer RNA** is a molecule that helps in the translation process, and is found in the cytoplasm.

Pairs of chromosomes are composed of DNA, which is tightly wound to conserve space. When replication starts, it unwinds. The steps in **DNA replication** are controlled by enzymes. The enzyme **helicase** instigates the deforming of hydrogen bonds between the bases to split the two strands. The splitting starts at the A-T bases (adenine and thymine) as there are only two hydrogen bonds. The cytosine-guanine base pair has three bonds. The term "**origin of replication**" is used to refer to where the splitting starts. The portion of the DNA that is unwound to be replicated is called the **replication fork**. Each strand of DNA is transcribed by an mRNA. It copies the DNA onto itself, base by base, in a complementary manner. The exception is that uracil replaces thymine.

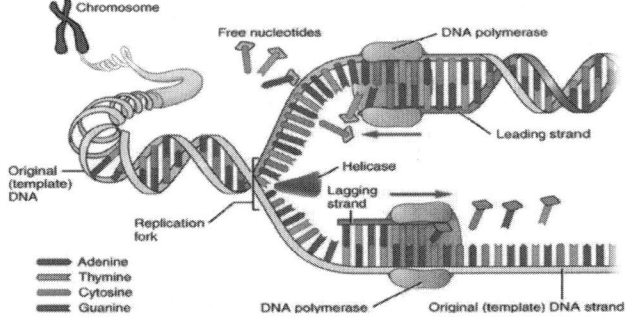

Science – Life and Physical Sciences
© Mometrix Media - flashcardsecrets.com/teas
ATI TEAS Exam

Differentiate between RNA and DNA.

Science – Life and Physical Sciences
© Mometrix Media - flashcardsecrets.com/teas
ATI TEAS Exam

Discuss Mendel's laws and Punnett squares.

Science – Life and Physical Sciences
© Mometrix Media - flashcardsecrets.com/teas
ATI TEAS Exam

Define and discuss gene, genotype, phenotype, and allele.

Science – Life and Physical Sciences
© Mometrix Media - flashcardsecrets.com/teas
ATI TEAS Exam

Discuss the concept of dominant and recessive.

Science – Life and Physical Sciences
© Mometrix Media - flashcardsecrets.com/teas
ATI TEAS Exam

Discuss genetic crosses, including monohybrid and dihybrid crosses.

Science – Life and Physical Sciences
© Mometrix Media - flashcardsecrets.com/teas
ATI TEAS Exam

Define and discuss a monohybrid cross.

Mendel's laws are the law of segregation (the first law), the law of independent assortment (the second law), and the law of dominance (the third law). The **law of segregation** states that there are two **alleles** and that half of the total number of alleles are contributed by each parent organism. The **law of independent assortment** states that traits are passed on randomly and are not influenced by other traits. The exception to this is linked traits. The **law of dominance** states that when two different alleles are present in a pair, the **dominant** one is expressed.

A **Punnett square** can illustrate how alleles combine from the contributing genes to form various **phenotypes**. One set of a parent's genes are put in columns, while the genes from the other parent are placed in rows. The allele combinations are shown in each cell. A Punnett square can be used to predict the outcome of crosses.

RNA and DNA differ in terms of structure and function. RNA has a different sugar than DNA. It has **ribose** rather than **deoxyribose** sugar. The RNA nitrogenous bases are adenine (A), guanine (G), cytosine (C), and uracil (U). **Uracil** is found only in RNA and **thymine** in found only in DNA. RNA consists of a single strand and DNA has two strands. If straightened out, DNA has two side rails. RNA only has one "backbone," or strand of sugar and phosphate group components. RNA uses the fully hydroxylated sugar **pentose**, which includes an extra oxygen compared to deoxyribose, which is the sugar used by DNA. RNA supports the functions carried out by DNA. It aids in gene expression, replication, and transportation.

Gene traits are represented in pairs with an uppercase letter for the dominant trait (A) and a lowercase letter for the recessive trait (a). Genes occur in pairs (AA, Aa, or aa). There is one gene on each chromosome half supplied by each parent organism. Since half the genetic material is from each parent, the offspring's traits are represented as a combination of these. A **dominant trait** only requires one gene of a gene pair for it to be expressed in a **phenotype**, whereas a **recessive** requires both genes in order to be manifested. For example, if the mother's genotype is Dd and the father's is dd, the possible combinations are Dd and dd. The dominant trait will be manifested if the genotype is DD or Dd. The recessive trait will be manifested if the genotype is dd. Both DD and dd are **homozygous** pairs. Dd is **heterozygous**.

A gene is a portion of DNA that identifies how traits are expressed and passed on in an organism. A gene is part of the **genetic code**. Collectively, all genes form the **genotype** of an individual. The genotype includes genes that may not be expressed, such as **recessive genes**. The **phenotype** is the physical, visual manifestation of genes. It is determined by the basic genetic information and how genes have been affected by their environment.

An **allele** is a variation of a gene. Also known as a trait, it determines the manifestation of a gene. This manifestation results in a specific physical appearance of some facet of an organism, such as eye color or height. For example, the genetic information for eye color is a gene. The gene variations responsible for blue, green, brown, or black eyes are called alleles. **Locus** (pl. loci) refers to the location of a gene or alleles.

A monohybrid cross is a genetic cross for a single trait that has two alleles. A monohybrid cross can be used to show which allele is **dominant** for a single trait. The first monohybrid cross typically occurs between two **homozygous** parents. Each parent is homozygous for a separate allele for a particular trait. For example, in pea plants, green pods (G) are dominant over yellow pods (g). In a genetic cross of two pea plants that are homozygous for pod color, the F_1 generation will be 100% heterozygous green pods.

	g	g
G	Gg	Gg
G	Gg	Gg

If the plants with the heterozygous green pods are crossed, the F_2 generation should be 50% heterozygous green, 25% homozygous green, and 25% homozygous yellow.

	G	g
G	GG	Gg
g	Gg	gg

Genetic crosses are the possible combinations of alleles, and can be represented using Punnett squares. A **monohybrid cross** refers to a cross involving only one trait. Typically, the ratio is 3:1 (DD, Dd, Dd, dd), which is the ratio of dominant gene manifestation to recessive gene manifestation. This ratio occurs when both parents have a pair of dominant and recessive genes. If one parent has a pair of dominant genes (DD) and the other has a pair of recessive (dd) genes, the recessive trait cannot be expressed in the next generation because the resulting crosses all have the Dd genotype.

A **dihybrid cross** refers to one involving more than one trait, which means more combinations are possible. The ratio of genotypes for a dihybrid cross is 9:3:3:1 when the traits are not linked. The ratio for incomplete dominance is 1:2:1, which corresponds to dominant, mixed, and recessive phenotypes.

Science – Life and Physical Sciences
ATI TEAS Exam

Define and discuss a dihybrid cross.

Science – Life and Physical Sciences
ATI TEAS Exam

Describe co-dominance and incomplete dominance.

Science – Life and Physical Sciences
ATI TEAS Exam

Describe polygenic inheritance and multiple alleles.

Science – Life and Physical Sciences
ATI TEAS Exam

Discuss atoms and their function.

Visit *mometrix.com/academy* for a related video.
Enter video code: 905932

Science – Life and Physical Sciences
ATI TEAS Exam

Discuss the size of atoms.

Science – Life and Physical Sciences
ATI TEAS Exam

Discuss atomic number and atomic mass.

Co-Dominance
Co-dominance refers to the expression of *both alleles* so that both traits are shown. Cows, for example, can have hair colors of red, white, or red and white (not pink). In the latter color, both traits are fully expressed. The ABO human blood typing system is also co-dominant.

Incomplete Dominance
Incomplete dominance is when both the **dominant** and **recessive** genes are expressed, resulting in a phenotype that is a mixture of the two. The fact that snapdragons can be red, white, or pink is a good example. The dominant red gene (RR) results in a red flower because of large amounts of red pigment. White (rr) occurs because both genes call for no pigment. Pink (Rr) occurs because one gene is for red and one is for no pigment. The colors blend to produce pink flowers. A cross of pink flowers (Rr) can result in red (RR), white (rr), or pink (Rr) flowers.

A dihybrid cross is a genetic cross for **two traits** that each have two alleles. For example, in pea plants, green pods (G) are dominant over yellow pods (g), and yellow seeds (Y) are dominant over green seeds (y). In a genetic cross of two pea plants that are homozygous for pod color and seed color, the F_1 generation will be 100% heterozygous green pods and yellow seeds (GgYy). If these F_1 plants are crossed, the resulting F_2 generation is shown below. There are nine genotypes for green-pod, yellow-seed plants: one GGYY, two GGYy, two GgYY, and four GgYy. There are three genotypes for green-pod, green-seed plants: one GGyy and two Ggyy. There are three genotypes for yellow-pod, yellow-seed plants: one ggYY and two ggYy. There is only one genotype for yellow-pod, green-seed plants: ggyy. This cross has a 9:3:3:1 ratio.

	GY	Gy	gY	gy
GY	GGYY	GGYy	GgYY	GgYy
Gy	GGYy	GGyy	GgYy	Ggyy
gY	GgYY	GgYy	ggYY	ggYy
gy	GgYy	Ggyy	ggYy	ggyy

All matter consists of atoms. Atoms consist of a **nucleus** and **electrons**. The nucleus consists of **protons** and **neutrons**. The properties of these are measurable; they have mass and an electrical charge. The nucleus is **positively charged** due to the presence of protons. Electrons are **negatively charged** and orbit the nucleus. The nucleus has considerably more mass than the surrounding electrons. Atoms can bond together to make **molecules**. Atoms that have an equal number of protons and electrons are electrically **neutral**. If the number of protons and electrons in an atom is not equal, the atom has a positive or negative charge and is an **ion**.

Polygenic Inheritance
Polygenic inheritance goes beyond the simplistic Mendelian concept that one gene influences one trait. It refers to traits that are influenced by *more than one gene*, and takes into account environmental influences on development.

Multiple Alleles
Each gene is made up of only two alleles, but in some cases, there are more than two possibilities for what those two alleles might be. For example, in blood typing, there are three alleles (A, B, O), but each person has only two of them. A gene with more than two possible alleles is known as a multiple allele. A gene that can result in two or more possible forms or expressions is known as a polymorphic gene.

Atomic Number
The atomic number of an element refers to the **number of protons** in the nucleus of an atom. It is a unique identifier. It can be represented as Z. Atoms with a neutral charge have an atomic number that is equal to the **number of electrons**.

Atomic Mass
Atomic mass is also known as the **mass number**. The atomic mass is the *total number of protons and neutrons* in the nucleus of an atom. It is referred to as "A." The atomic mass (A) is equal to the number of protons (Z) plus the number of neutrons (N). This can be represented by the equation $A = Z + N$. The mass of electrons in an atom is basically insignificant because it is so small. Atomic weight may sometimes be referred to as "**relative atomic mass**," but should not be confused with atomic mass. Atomic weight is the ratio of the average mass per atom of a sample (which can include various isotopes of an element) to 1/12 of the mass of an atom of carbon-12.

Atoms are extremely small. A hydrogen atom is about 5×10^{-8} mm in diameter. According to some estimates, five trillion hydrogen atoms could fit on the head of a pin. **Atomic radius** refers to the average distance between the nucleus and the outermost electron. Models of atoms that include the proton, nucleus, and electrons typically show the electrons very close to the nucleus and revolving around it, similar to how the Earth orbits the sun. However, another model relates the Earth as the nucleus and its atmosphere as electrons, which is the basis of the term "**electron cloud**." Another description is that electrons swarm around the nucleus. It should be noted that these atomic models are not to scale. A more accurate representation would be a nucleus with a diameter of about 2 cm in a stadium. The electrons would be in the bleachers. This model is similar to the not-to-scale solar system model. In reference to the periodic table, atomic radius increases as energy levels are added and decreases as more protons are added (because they pull the electrons closer to the nucleus). Essentially, atomic radius increases toward the left and toward the bottom of the periodic table (i.e., Francium (Fr) has the largest atomic radius while Helium (He) has the smallest).

Science – Life and Physical Sciences
© Mometrix Media - flashcardsecrets.com/teas
ATI TEAS Exam

Describe isotopes and their functions.

Science – Life and Physical Sciences
© Mometrix Media - flashcardsecrets.com/teas
ATI TEAS Exam

Describe electrons and their functions.

Science – Life and Physical Sciences
© Mometrix Media - flashcardsecrets.com/teas
ATI TEAS Exam

Discuss chemical bonds.

Science – Life and Physical Sciences
© Mometrix Media - flashcardsecrets.com/teas
ATI TEAS Exam

Discuss the charges of atoms.

Science – Life and Physical Sciences
© Mometrix Media - flashcardsecrets.com/teas
ATI TEAS Exam

Describe bonding between atoms.

Science – Life and Physical Sciences
© Mometrix Media - flashcardsecrets.com/teas
ATI TEAS Exam

Explain the different chemical bonds between atoms.

Electrons are subatomic particles that orbit the nucleus at various levels commonly referred to as **layers, shells,** or **clouds**. The orbiting electron or electrons account for only a fraction of the atom's mass. They are much smaller than the nucleus, are negatively charged, and exhibit wave-like characteristics. Electrons are part of the **lepton** family of elementary particles. Electrons can occupy orbits that are varying distances away from the nucleus, and tend to occupy the lowest energy level they can. If an atom has all its electrons in the lowest available positions, it has a **stable** electron arrangement. The outermost electron shell of an atom in its uncombined state is known as the **valence shell**. The electrons there are called **valence electrons**, and it is their number that determines **bonding behavior**. Atoms tend to react in a manner that will allow them to fill or empty their valence shells.

Isotopes are atoms of the same element that vary in their number of neutrons. Isotopes of the same element have the same number of protons and thus the same atomic number. They are denoted by the element symbol, preceded in superscript and subscript by the mass number and atomic number, respectively. For instance, the notations for protium, deuterium, and tritium are, respectively: $_1^1H$, $_1^2H$, and $_1^3H$.

Isotopes that have not been observed to decay are **stable**, or non-radioactive, isotopes. It is not known whether some stable isotopes may have such long decay times that observing decay is not possible. Currently, 80 elements have one or more stable isotopes. There are 256 known stable isotopes in total. Carbon, for example, has three isotopes. Two (carbon-12 and carbon-13) are stable and one (carbon-14) is radioactive. **Radioactive isotopes** have unstable nuclei and can undergo spontaneous nuclear reactions, which results in particles or radiation being emitted. It cannot be predicted when a specific nucleus will decay, but large groups of identical nuclei decay at predictable rates. Knowledge about rates of decay can be used to *estimate the age of materials* that contain radioactive isotopes.

Most atoms are **neutral** since the positive charge of the protons in the nucleus is balanced by the negative charge of the surrounding electrons. Electrons are transferred between atoms when they come into contact with each other. This creates a molecule or atom in which the number of electrons does not equal the number of protons, which gives it a positive or negative charge. A **negative ion** is created when an atom gains electrons, while a **positive ion** is created when an atom loses electrons. An **ionic bond** is formed between ions with opposite charges. The resulting compound is neutral. **Ionization** refers to the process by which neutral particles are ionized into charged particles. Gases and plasmas can be partially or fully ionized through ionization.

Chemical bonds involve a negative-positive attraction between an electron or electrons and the nucleus of an atom or nuclei of more than one atom. The attraction keeps the atom cohesive, but also enables the formation of bonds among other atoms and molecules. Each of the four **energy levels** (or shells) of an atom has a maximum number of electrons they can contain. Each level must be completely filled before electrons can be added to the **valence level**. The farther away from the nucleus an electron is, the more energy it has. The first shell, or K-shell, can hold a maximum of 2 electrons; the second, the L-shell, can hold 8; the third, the M-shell, can hold 18; the fourth, the N-shell, can hold 32. The shells can also have **subshells**. Chemical bonds form and break between atoms when atoms gain, lose, or share an electron in the outer valence shell. **Polar bond** refers to a covalent type of bond with a separation of charge. One end is negative and the other is positive. The hydrogen-oxygen bond in water is one example of a polar bond.

A union between the electron structures of atoms is called **chemical bonding**. An atom may gain, surrender, or share its electrons with another atom it bonds with. Listed below are three types of chemical bonding.

- **Ionic bonding** – When an atom gains or loses electrons it becomes negatively or positively charged, turning it into an ion. An ionic bond is a relationship between two *oppositely charged ions*.
- **Covalent bonding** – Atoms that share electrons have what is called a covalent bond. Electrons shared equally have a *non-polar bond*, while electrons shared unequally have a *polar bond*.
- **Hydrogen bonding** – The atom of a molecule interacts with a hydrogen atom in the same area. Hydrogen bonds can also form between two different parts of the same molecule, as in the structure of DNA and other large molecules.

A **cation** or positive ion is formed when an atom loses one or more electrons. An **anion** or negative ion is formed when an atom gains one or more electrons.

Atoms of the same element may bond together to form **molecules** or **crystalline solids**. When two or more different types of atoms bind together chemically, a **compound** is made. The physical properties of compounds reflect the nature of the interactions among their molecules. These interactions are determined by the structure of the molecule, including the atoms they consist of and the distances and angles between them.

Explain ionic bonding.

Explain covalent bonding.

Describe electronegativity with atoms.

Discuss the basic organization of matter.

Explain the periodic table of elements and it's organization.

Describe the periodic table.

Covalent bonding is characterized by the sharing of one or more pairs of electrons between two atoms or between an atom and another **covalent bond**. This produces an attraction to repulsion stability that holds these molecules together.

Atoms have the tendency to share electrons with each other so that all outer electron shells are filled. The resultant bonds are always stronger than the **intermolecular hydrogen bond** and are similar in strength to ionic bonds.

Covalent bonding occurs most frequently between atoms with similar **electronegativities**. **Nonmetals** are more likely to form covalent bonds than metals since it is more difficult for nonmetals to liberate an electron. **Electron sharing** takes place when one species encounters another species with similar electronegativity. Covalent bonding of metals is important in both *process chemistry* and *industrial catalysis*.

The transfer of electrons from one atom to another is called **ionic bonding**. Atoms that lose or gain electrons are referred to as **ions**. The gain or loss of electrons will result in an ion having a positive or negative charge. Here is an example:

Take an atom of sodium (Na) and an atom of chlorine (Cl). The sodium atom has a total of 11 electrons (including one electron in its outer shell). The chlorine has 17 electrons (including 7 electrons in its outer shell). From this, the atomic number, or number of protons, of sodium can be calculated as 11 because the number of protons equals the number of electrons in an atom. When sodium chloride (NaCl) is formed, one electron from sodium transfers to chlorine. Ions have charges. They are written with a plus (+) or minus (−) symbol. Ions in a compound are attracted to each other because they have *opposite charges*.

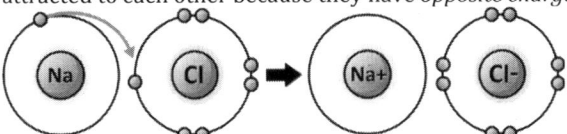

An **element** is the most basic type of matter. It has unique properties and cannot be broken down into other elements. The smallest unit of an element is the **atom**. A chemical combination of two or more types of elements is called a **compound**.

Compounds often have properties that are very different from those of their constituent elements. The smallest independent unit of an element or compound is known as a **molecule**. Most elements are found somewhere in nature in single-atom form, but a few elements only exist naturally in pairs. These are called **diatomic elements**, of which some of the most common are hydrogen, nitrogen, and oxygen.

Elements and compounds are represented by **chemical symbols**, one or two letters, most often the first in the element name. More than one atom of the same element in a compound is represented with a subscript number designating how many atoms of that element are present. Water, for instance, contains two hydrogens and one oxygen. Thus, the chemical formula is H_2O. Methane contains one carbon and four hydrogens, so its formula is CH_4.

Electronegativity is a measure of how capable an atom is of attracting a pair of bonding electrons. It refers to the fact that one atom exerts slightly more force in a bond than another, creating a **dipole**. If the electronegative difference between two atoms is small, the atoms will form a **polar covalent bond**. If the difference is large, the atoms will form an **ionic bond**. When there is no electronegativity, a **pure nonpolar covalent bond** is formed.

A typical periodic table shows the elements' symbols and atomic number, the number of protons in the atomic nucleus. Some more detailed tables also list **atomic mass**, **electronegativity**, and other data. The position of an element in the table reveals its group, its block, and whether it is a representative, transition, or inner transition element. Its position also shows the element as a metal, nonmetal, or metalloid.

For the representative elements, the last digit of the **group number** reveals the number of outer-level electrons. Roman numerals for the A groups also reveal the number of outer level electrons within the group. The position of the element in the table reveals its **electronic configuration** and how it differs in atomic size from neighbors in its period or group. In this example, Boron has an atomic number of 5 and an atomic weight of 10.811. It is found in group 13, in which all atoms of the group have 3 valence electrons; the group's Roman numeral representation is IIIA.

The **periodic table** is a tabular arrangement of the elements and is organized according to **periodic law**. The properties of the elements depend on their **atomic structure** and vary with **atomic number**. It shows periodic trends of physical and chemical properties and identifies families of elements with similar properties. In the periodic table, the elements are arranged by atomic number in horizontal rows called **periods** and vertical columns called **groups** or **families**. They are further categorized as metals, metalloids, or nonmetals. The majority of known elements are metals; there are seventeen nonmetals and eight metalloids. **Metals** are situated at the left end of the periodic table, **nonmetals** to the right and **metalloids** between the two.

Discuss the important features of the periodic table and its structure.

Define and discuss chemical reactivity in terms of the periodic table.

Discuss the significance of groups and periods in terms of reactivity.

Discuss metals on the periodic table.

Describe intensive and extensive properties.

Describe physical properties and how they can be observed and measured.

Visit *mometrix.com/academy* for a related video.
Enter video code: 920570

Reactivity refers to the tendency of a substance to engage in **chemical reactions**. If that tendency is high, the substance is said to be highly reactive, or to have **high reactivity**. Because the basis of a chemical reaction is the transfer of electrons, reactivity depends upon the presence of uncommitted electrons which are available for transfer. **Periodicity** allows us to predict an element's reactivity based on its position on the periodic table. High numbered groups on the right side of the table have a fuller complement of electrons in their outer levels, making them less likely to react. Noble gases, on the far right of the table, each have eight electrons in the outer level, with the exception of He, which has two. Because atoms tend to lose or gain electrons to reach an ideal of eight in the outer level, these elements have very low reactivity.

The most important feature of the table is its arrangement according to **periodicity**, or the predictable trends observable in atoms. The arrangement enables classification, organization, and prediction of important elemental properties.

The table is organized in horizontal rows called **Periods**, and vertical columns called **Groups** or **Families**. Groups of elements share predictable characteristics, the most important of which is that their outer energy levels have the same configuration of electrons. For example, the highest group is group 18, the noble gases. Each element in this group has a full complement of electrons in its outer level, making the reactivity low. Elements in periods also share some common properties, but most classifications rely more heavily on groups.

The metals are located on the left side and center of the periodic table, and the nonmetals are located on the right side of the periodic table. The metalloids or semimetals form a zigzag line between the metals and nonmetals. Metals include the **alkali metals** such as lithium, sodium, and potassium and the **alkaline earth metals** such as beryllium, magnesium, and calcium. Metals also include the **transition metals** such as iron, copper, and nickel and the **inner transition metals** such as thorium, uranium, and plutonium. **Nonmetals** include the **chalcogens** such as oxygen and sulfur, the **halogens** such as fluorine and chlorine, and the **noble gases** such as helium and argon. Carbon, nitrogen, and phosphorus are also nonmetals. **Metalloids** or **semimetals** include boron, silicon, germanium, antimony, and polonium.

Reading left to right within a period, each element contains one more electron than the one preceding it. (Note that H and He are in the same period, though nothing is between them and they are in different groups.) As electrons are added, their attraction to the nucleus increases, meaning that as we read to the right in a period, each atom's electrons are more densely compacted, more strongly bound to the nucleus, and less likely to be pulled away in reactions. As we read down a group, each successive atom's outer electrons are less tightly bound to the nucleus, thus increasing their reactivity, because the principal energy levels are increasingly full as we move downward within the group. **Principal energy levels** shield the outer energy levels from nuclear attraction, allowing the valence electrons to react. For this reason, noble gases farther down the group can react under certain circumstances.

Physical properties are any property of matter that can be **observed** or **measured**. These include properties such as color, elasticity, mass, volume, and temperature. **Mass** is a measure of the amount of substance in an object. **Weight** is a measure of the gravitational pull of Earth on an object. **Volume** is a measure of the amount of space occupied. There are many formulas to determine volume. For example, the volume of a cube is the length of one side cubed (a^3) and the volume of a rectangular prism is length times width times height ($l \times w \times h$). The volume of an irregular shape can be determined by how much water it displaces. **Density** is a measure of the amount of mass per unit volume. The formula to find density is mass divided by volume ($D=m/V$). It is expressed in terms of mass per cubic unit, such as grams per cubic centimeter (g/cm^3). **Specific gravity** is a measure of the ratio of a substance's density compared to the density of water.

Physical properties are categorized as either intensive or extensive. **Intensive properties** *do not* depend on the amount of matter or quantity of the sample. This means that intensive properties will not change if the sample size is increased or decreased. Intensive properties include color, hardness, melting point, boiling point, density, ductility, malleability, specific heat, temperature, concentration, and magnetization.

Extensive properties *do* depend on the amount of matter or quantity of the sample. Therefore, extensive properties do change if the sample size is increased or decreased. If the sample size is increased, the property increases. If the sample size is decreased, the property decreases. Extensive properties include volume, mass, weight, energy, entropy, number of moles, and electrical charge.

Science – Life and Physical Sciences
© Mometrix Media - flashcardsecrets.com/teas
ATI TEAS Exam

Discuss density and specific heat capacity.

Visit *mometrix.com/academy* for a related video.
Enter video code: 736791

Science – Life and Physical Sciences
© Mometrix Media - flashcardsecrets.com/teas
ATI TEAS Exam

Describe the flow of heat.

Science – Life and Physical Sciences
© Mometrix Media - flashcardsecrets.com/teas
ATI TEAS Exam

Explain the difference between the physical and chemical properties of matter.

Science – Life and Physical Sciences
© Mometrix Media - flashcardsecrets.com/teas
ATI TEAS Exam

Discuss the unique properties of water.

Visit *mometrix.com/academy* for a related video.
Enter video code: 279526

Science – Life and Physical Sciences
© Mometrix Media - flashcardsecrets.com/teas
ATI TEAS Exam

Describe hydrogen bonds and how they're formed.

Science – Life and Physical Sciences
© Mometrix Media - flashcardsecrets.com/teas
ATI TEAS Exam

Identify and discuss the various passive transport mechanisms used by cells.

Heat always flows from a region of higher temperature to a region of lower temperature. If two regions are at the same temperature, there is a **thermal equilibrium** between them and there will be **no net heat transfer** between them. **Conduction** is a form of heat transfer that requires contact. Since heat is a measure of kinetic energy, most commonly vibration, at the atomic level, it may be transferred from one location to another or one object to another by contact.

Density
The density of an object is equal to its *mass divided by its volume* (d = m/v). It is important to note the difference between an *object's density* and a *material's density*. Water has a density of one gram per cubic centimeter, while steel has a density approximately eight times that. Despite having a much higher material density, an object made of steel may still float. A hollow steel sphere, for instance, will float easily because the density of the object includes the air contained within the sphere.

Specific Heat Capacity
Specific heat capacity, also known as **specific heat**, is the *heat capacity per unit mass*. Each element and compound has its own specific heat. For example, it takes different amounts of heat energy to raise the temperature of the same amounts of magnesium and lead by one degree. The equation for relating heat energy to specific heat capacity is $Q = mc\Delta T$, where m represents the mass of the object, and c represents its specific heat capacity.

The important properties of water (H$_2$O) are *high polarity, hydrogen bonding, cohesiveness, adhesiveness, high specific heat, high latent heat, and high heat of vaporization*. It is **essential to life** as we know it, as water is one of the main if not the main constituent of many living things. Water is a liquid at room temperature. The high specific heat of water means it resists the breaking of its hydrogen bonds and resists heat and motion, which is why it has a relatively high boiling point and high vaporization point. It also resists temperature change. In its solid state, water floats. (Most substances are heavier in their solid forms.) Water is **cohesive**, which means it is attracted to itself. It is also **adhesive**, which means it readily attracts other molecules. If water tends to adhere to another substance, the substance is said to be **hydrophilic**. Because of its cohesive and adhesive properties, water makes a good solvent. Substances, particularly those with polar ions and molecules, readily dissolve in water.

If a chemical change must be carried out in order to observe and measure a property, then the property is a **chemical property**. For example, when hydrogen gas is burned in oxygen, it forms water. This is a chemical property of hydrogen because after burning, a different chemical substance – water – is all that remains. The hydrogen cannot be recovered from the water by means of a physical change such as freezing or boiling.

Transport mechanisms allow for the movement of substances through membranes. **Passive transport mechanisms** include simple and facilitated diffusion and osmosis. They do not require energy from the cell. **Diffusion** occurs when particles are transported from areas of higher concentration to areas of lower concentration. When equilibrium is reached, diffusion stops. Examples are gas exchange (carbon dioxide and oxygen) during photosynthesis and the transport of oxygen from air to blood and from blood to tissue. **Facilitated diffusion** occurs when specific molecules are transported by a specific carrier protein. **Carrier proteins** vary in terms of size, shape, and charge. Glucose and amino acids are examples of substances transported by carrier proteins.

Osmosis is the diffusion of water through a semi-permeable membrane from an area of lower solute concentration to one of higher solute concentration. Examples of osmosis include the absorption of water by plant roots and the alimentary canal. Plants lose and gain water through osmosis. A plant cell that swells because of water retention is said to be **turgid**.

Hydrogen bonds are weaker than covalent and ionic bonds, and refer to the type of attraction in an **electronegative atom** such as oxygen, fluorine, or nitrogen. Hydrogen bonds can form within a single molecule or between molecules. A water molecule is **polar**, meaning it is partially positively charged on one end (the hydrogen end) and partially negatively charged on the other (the oxygen end). This is because the hydrogen atoms are arranged around the oxygen atom in a close tetrahedron. Hydrogen is **oxidized** (its number of electrons is reduced) when it bonds with oxygen to form water. Hydrogen bonds tend not only to be weak but also short-lived. They also tend to be numerous. Hydrogen bonds give water many of its important properties, including its high specific heat and high heat of vaporization, its solvent qualities, its adhesiveness and cohesiveness, its hydrophilic qualities, and its ability to float in its solid form. Hydrogen bonds are also an important component of *proteins, nucleic acids, and DNA*.

Define matter and discuss the three states of matter.

Outline the characteristic properties of gases, liquids, and solids.

Discuss the process of matter moving from one state to another and the role of heat in the process.

Visit *mometrix.com/academy* for a related video.
Enter video code: 742449

Discuss the names given to the six different types of phase change.

Explain the process of evaporation.

Explain the process of condensation.

The table below outlines the characteristic properties of the three states of matter:

State of matter	Volume/shape	Density	Compressibility	Molecular motion
Gas	Assumes volume and shape of its container	Low	High	Very free motion
Liquid	Volume remains constant but it assumes shape of its container	High	Virtually none	Move past each other freely
Solid	Definite volume and shape	High	Virtually none	Vibrate around fixed positions

Matter refers to substances that *have mass and occupy space* (or volume). The traditional definition of matter describes it as having three states: solid, liquid, and gas. These different states are caused by differences in the distances and angles between molecules or atoms, which result in differences in the energy that binds them. **Solid** structures are rigid or nearly rigid and have strong bonds. Molecules or atoms of **liquids** move around and have weak bonds, although they are not weak enough to readily break. Molecules or atoms of **gases** move almost independently of each other, are typically far apart, and do not form bonds. The current definition of matter describes it as having four states. The fourth is **plasma**, which is an ionized gas that has some electrons that are described as free because they are not bound to an atom or molecule. However, the TEAS will only be concerned with solids, liquids, and gases.

A substance that is undergoing a change from a solid to a liquid is said to be **melting**. If this change occurs in the opposite direction, from liquid to solid, this change is called **freezing**. A liquid which is being converted to a gas is undergoing **vaporization**. The reverse of this process is known as **condensation**. Direct transitions from gas to solid and solid to gas are much less common in everyday life, but they can occur given the proper conditions. Solid to gas conversion is known as **sublimation**, while the reverse is called **deposition**.

The three states of matter can be traversed by the addition or removal of **heat**. For example, when a solid is heated to its melting point, it can begin to form a liquid. However, in order to transition from solid to liquid, additional heat must be added at the melting point to overcome the **latent heat of fusion**. Upon further heating to its boiling point, the liquid can begin to form a gas, but again, additional heat must be added at the boiling point to overcome the **latent heat of vaporization**.

In the solid state, water is less dense than in the liquid state. This can be observed quite simply by noting that an ice cube floats at the surface of a glass of water. Were this not the case, ice would not form on the surface of lakes and rivers in those regions of the world where the climate produces temperatures below the freezing point. If water behaved as other substances do, lakes and rivers would freeze from the bottom up, which would be detrimental to many forms of aquatic life.

The lower density of ice occurs because of a combination of the unique structure of the water molecule and hydrogen bonding. In the case of ice, each oxygen atom is bound to four hydrogen atoms, two covalently and two by hydrogen bonds. This forms an ordered roughly **tetrahedral** structure that prevents the molecules from getting close to each other. As such, there are empty spaces in the structure that account for the low density of ice.

Condensation is the phase change in a substance from a gaseous to liquid form; it is the opposite of evaporation or vaporization. When temperatures decrease in a gas, such as water vapor, the material's component molecules move more slowly. The decreased motion of the molecules enables **intermolecular cohesive forces** to pull the molecules closer together and, in water, establish hydrogen bonds. Condensation can also be caused by an increase in the pressure exerted on a gas, which results in a decrease in the substance's volume (it reduces the distance between particles). In the **hydrologic cycle**, this process is initiated when warm air containing water vapor rises and then cools. This occurs due to convection in the air, meteorological fronts, or lifting over high land formations.

Evaporation: Evaporation is the change of state in a substance from a liquid to a gaseous form at a temperature below its boiling point (the temperature at which all of the molecules in a liquid are changed to gas through vaporization). Some of the molecules at the surface of a liquid always maintain enough **heat energy** to escape the cohesive forces exerted on them by neighboring molecules. At higher temperatures, the molecules in a substance move more rapidly, increasing their number with enough energy to break out of the liquid form. The rate of evaporation is higher when more of the surface area of a liquid is exposed (as in a large water body, such as an ocean). The amount of moisture already in the air also affects the rate of evaporation—if there is a significant amount of water vapor in the air around a liquid, some evaporated molecules will return to the liquid. The speed of the evaporation process is also decreased by increased **atmospheric pressure**.

Provide a general overview of chemical reactions.

Explain how to read chemical equations.

List some methods for balancing equations.

Define the Law of Conservation of Mass and how it relates to chemical reactions.

Discuss the basic mechanisms of chemical reactions.

Define and discuss combination reactions.

Chemical equations describe chemical reactions. The **reactants** are on the left side before the arrow and the **products** are on the right side after the arrow. The arrow indicates the **reaction** or change. The **coefficient**, or stoichiometric coefficient, is the number before the element, and indicates the ratio of reactants to products in terms of moles. The equation for the formation of water from hydrogen and oxygen, for example, is $2H_{2(g)} + O_{2(g)} \rightarrow 2H_2O_{(l)}$. The 2 preceding hydrogen and water is the coefficient, which means there are 2 moles of hydrogen and 2 of water. There is 1 mole of oxygen, which does not have to be indicated with the number 1. In parentheses, *g* stands for gas, *l* stands for liquid, *s* stands for solid, and *aq* stands for aqueous solution (a substance dissolved in water). **Charges** are shown in superscript for individual ions, but not for ionic compounds. **Polyatomic ions** are separated by parentheses so the ion will not be confused with the number of ions.

Chemical reactions measured in human time can take place quickly or slowly. They can take a fraction of a second or billions of years. The **rates** of chemical reactions are determined by how frequently reacting atoms and molecules interact. Rates are also influenced by the temperature and various properties (such as shape) of the reacting materials. **Catalysts** accelerate chemical reactions, while **inhibitors** decrease reaction rates. Some types of reactions release energy in the form of heat and light. Some types of reactions involve the transfer of either electrons or hydrogen ions between reacting ions, molecules, or atoms. In other reactions, chemical bonds are broken down by heat or light to form **reactive radicals** with electrons that will readily form new bonds. Processes such as the formation of ozone and greenhouse gases in the atmosphere and the burning and processing of fossil fuels are controlled by radical reactions.

The Law of Conservation of Mass in a chemical reaction is commonly stated as follows:

In a chemical reaction, matter is neither created nor destroyed.

What this means is that there will always be the same **total mass** of material after a reaction as before. This allows for predicting how molecules will combine by balanced equations in which the number of each type of atom is the same on either side of the equation. For example, two hydrogen molecules combine with one oxygen molecule to form water. This is a balanced chemical equation because the number of each type of atom is the same on both sides of the arrow. It has to balance because the reaction obeys the Law of Conservation of Mass.

An **unbalanced equation** is one that does not follow the **law of conservation of mass**, which states that matter can only be changed, not created. If an equation is unbalanced, the numbers of atoms indicated by the stoichiometric coefficients on each side of the arrow will not be equal. Start by writing the formulas for each species in the reaction. Count the atoms on each side and determine if the number is equal. Coefficients must be whole numbers. Fractional amounts, such as half a molecule, are not possible. Equations can be balanced by multiplying the coefficients by a constant that will produce the smallest possible whole number coefficient. $H_2 + O_2 \rightarrow H_2O$ is an example of an unbalanced equation. The balanced equation is $2H_2 + O_2 \rightarrow 2H_2O$, which indicates that it takes two moles of hydrogen and one of oxygen to produce two moles of water.

Combination Reactions
Combination, or synthesis, reactions: In a combination reaction, two or more reactants combine to make one product. This can be seen in the equation A + B → AB. These reactions are also called **synthesis** or **addition reactions**. An example is burning hydrogen in air to produce water. The equation is $2H_2 (g) + O_2 (g) \rightarrow 2H_2O (l)$. Another example is when water and sulfur trioxide react to form sulfuric acid. The equation is $H_2O + SO_3 \rightarrow H_2SO_4$.

Chemical reactions normally occur when electrons are transferred from one atom or molecule to another. Reactions and reactivity depend on the **octet rule**, which describes the tendency of atoms to gain or lose electrons until their outer energy levels contain eight. The changes in a reaction may be in **composition** or **configuration** of a compound or substance, and result in one or more products being generated which were not present in isolation before the reaction occurred. For instance, when oxygen reacts with methane (CH_4), water and carbon dioxide are the products; one set of substances (CH_4 + O) was transformed into a new set of substances (CO_2 + H_2O).

Reactions depend on the presence of a **reactant**, or substance undergoing change, a **reagent**, or partner in the reaction less transformed than the reactant (such as a catalyst), and **products**, or the final result of the reaction. **Reaction conditions**, or environmental factors, are also important components in reactions. These include conditions such as temperature, pressure, concentration, whether the reaction occurs in solution, the type of solution, and presence or absence of catalysts. Chemical reactions are usually written in the following format: Reactants → Products.

Science – Life and Physical Sciences
ATI TEAS Exam

Define and discuss decomposition reactions.

Science – Life and Physical Sciences
ATI TEAS Exam

Discuss single substitution, displacement, and replacement reactions.

Visit *mometrix.com/academy* for a related video.
Enter video code: 442975

Science – Life and Physical Sciences
ATI TEAS Exam

Explain metathesis (acid/base) reactions.

Science – Life and Physical Sciences
ATI TEAS Exam

Define and discuss combustion.

Visit *mometrix.com/academy* for a related video.
Enter video code: 592219

Science – Life and Physical Sciences
ATI TEAS Exam

Explain the effects of catalysts on reactions and define the Maxwell-Boltzmann distribution.

Science – Life and Physical Sciences
ATI TEAS Exam

Define pH and discuss the pH scale.

Visit *mometrix.com/academy* for a related video.
Enter video code: 187395

Single substitution, displacement, or replacement reactions occur when one reactant is displaced by another to form the final product (A + BC → B + AC). Single substitution reactions can be **cationic** or **anionic**. When a piece of copper (Cu) is placed into a solution of silver nitrate ($AgNO_3$), the solution turns blue. The copper appears to be replaced with a silvery-white material. The equation is $2AgNO_3 + Cu \rightarrow Cu(NO_3)_2 + 2Ag$. When this reaction takes place, the copper dissolves and the silver in the silver nitrate solution precipitates (becomes a solid), thus resulting in copper nitrate and silver. Copper and silver have switched places in the nitrate.

Decomposition (or desynthesis, decombination, or deconstruction) reactions; in a decomposition reaction, a reactant is broken down into two or more products. This can be seen in the equation AB → A + B. When a compound or substance separates into these simpler substances, the **byproducts** are often substances that are different from the original. Decomposition can be viewed as the *opposite* of combination reactions. These reactions are also called analysis reactions. Most decomposition reactions are **endothermic**. Heat needs to be added for the chemical reaction to occur. **Thermal decomposition** is caused by heat. **Electrolytic decomposition** is due to electricity. An example of this type of reaction is the decomposition of water into hydrogen and oxygen gas. The equation is $2H_2O \rightarrow 2H_2 + O_2$. Separation processes can be **mechanical** or **chemical**, and usually involve reorganizing a mixture of substances without changing their chemical nature. The separated products may differ from the original mixture in terms of chemical or physical properties. Types of separation processes include **filtration**, **crystallization**, **distillation**, and **chromatography**. Basically, decomposition *breaks down* one compound into two or more compounds or substances that are different from the original; separation *sorts* the substances from the original mixture into like substances.

Combustion, or burning, is a sequence of chemical reactions involving **fuel** and an **oxidant** that produces heat and sometimes light. There are many types of combustion, such as rapid, slow, complete, turbulent, microgravity, and incomplete. Fuels and oxidants determine the **compounds** formed by a combustion reaction. For example, when rocket fuel consisting of hydrogen and oxygen combusts, it results in the formation of water vapor. When air and wood burn, resulting compounds include nitrogen, unburned carbon, and carbon compounds. Combustion is an **exothermic** process, meaning it releases energy. Exothermic energy is commonly released as heat, but can take other forms, such as light, electricity, or sound.

Double displacement, double replacement, substitution, metathesis, or ion exchange reactions occur when ions or bonds are exchanged by two compounds to form different compounds (AC + BD → AD + BC). An example of this is that silver nitrate and sodium chloride form two different products (silver chloride and sodium nitrate) when they react. The formula for this reaction is $AgNO_3 + NaCl \rightarrow AgCl + NaNO_3$.

Double replacement reactions are **metathesis reactions**. In a double replacement reaction, the chemical reactants exchange ions but the oxidation state stays the same. One of the indicators of this is the formation of a **solid precipitate**. In acid/base reactions, an **acid** is a compound that can donate a proton, while a **base** is a compound that can accept a proton. In these types of reactions, the acid and base react to form a salt and water. When the proton is donated, the base becomes **water** and the remaining ions form a **salt**. One method of determining whether a reaction is an oxidation/reduction or a metathesis reaction is that the oxidation number of atoms does not change during a metathesis reaction.

The **potential of hydrogen** (pH) is a measurement of the *concentration of hydrogen ions* in a substance in terms of the number of moles of H^+ per liter of solution. All substances fall between 0 and 14 on the pH scale. A lower pH indicates a higher H^+ concentration, while a higher pH indicates a lower H^+ concentration.

Pure water has a **neutral pH**, which is 7. Anything with a pH lower than pure water (<7) is considered **acidic**. Anything with a pH higher than pure water (>7) is a **base**. Drain cleaner, soap, baking soda, ammonia, egg whites, and sea water are common bases. Urine, stomach acid, citric acid, vinegar, hydrochloric acid, and battery acid are acids. A **pH indicator** is a substance that acts as a detector of hydrogen or hydronium ions. It is **halochromic**, meaning it changes color to indicate that hydrogen or hydronium ions have been detected.

Catalysts, substances that help *change the rate of reaction* without changing their form, can increase reaction rate by decreasing the number of steps it takes to form products. The **mass** of the catalyst should be the same at the beginning of the reaction as it is at the end. The **activation energy** is the minimum amount required to get a reaction started. Activation energy causes particles to collide with sufficient energy to start the reaction. A **catalyst** enables more particles to react, which lowers the activation energy. Examples of catalysts in reactions are manganese oxide (MnO_2) in the decomposition of hydrogen peroxide, iron in the manufacture of ammonia using the Haber process, and concentrate of sulfuric acid in the nitration of benzene.

Science – Life and Physical Sciences
© Mometrix Media - flashcardsecrets.com/teas
ATI TEAS Exam

Defined bases and discuss their observable properties.

Science – Life and Physical Sciences
© Mometrix Media - flashcardsecrets.com/teas
ATI TEAS Exam

Discuss physical properties of acids.

Science – Life and Physical Sciences
© Mometrix Media - flashcardsecrets.com/teas
ATI TEAS Exam

Define what is meant by the descriptions of acids and bases as strong or weak.

Visit *mometrix.com/academy* for a related video.
Enter video code: 268930

Science – Life and Physical Sciences
© Mometrix Media - flashcardsecrets.com/teas
ATI TEAS Exam

Describe properties of salts and how they're formed.

Science – Scientific Reasoning
© Mometrix Media - flashcardsecrets.com/teas
ATI TEAS Exam

Discuss the metric system and the basic units of measurement.

Science – Scientific Reasoning
© Mometrix Media - flashcardsecrets.com/teas
ATI TEAS Exam

Describe how SI is measured.

Acids are a unique class of compounds characterized by consistent properties. The most significant property of an acid is not readily observable and is what gives acids their unique behaviors: the **ionization of H atoms**, or their tendency to dissociate from their parent molecules and take on an electrical charge. **Carboxylic acids** are also characterized by ionization, but of the O atoms. Some other properties of acids are easy to observe without any experimental apparatus. These properties include the following:

- They have a sour taste
- They change the color of litmus paper to red
- They produce gaseous H_2 in reaction with some metals
- They produce salt precipitates in reaction with bases

Other properties, while no more complex, are less easily observed. For instance, most inorganic acids are easily soluble in water and have high boiling points.

Basic chemicals are usually in aqueous solution and have the following traits: a bitter taste; a soapy or slippery texture to the touch; the capacity to restore the blue color of litmus paper which had previously been turned red by an acid; the ability to produce salts in reaction with acids. The word **alkaline** is used to describe bases.

In contrast to acids, which yield **hydrogen ions** (H^+) when dissolved in solution, bases yield **hydroxide ions** (OH^-); the same models used to describe acids can be inverted and used to describe bases—Arrhenius, Bronsted-Lowry, and Lewis.

Some **nonmetal oxides** (such as Na_2O) are classified as bases even though they do not contain hydroxides in their molecular form. However, these substances easily produce hydroxide ions when reacted with water, which is why they are classified as bases.

Some properties of **salts** are that they are formed from acid base reactions, are ionic compounds consisting of metallic and nonmetallic ions, dissociate in water, and are comprised of tightly bonded ions. Some common salts are sodium chloride (NaCl), sodium bisulfate, potassium dichromate ($K_2Cr_2O_7$), and calcium chloride ($CaCl_2$). Calcium chloride is used as a drying agent, and may be used to absorb moisture when freezing mixtures. Potassium nitrate (KNO_3) is used to make fertilizer and in the manufacture of explosives. Sodium nitrate ($NaNO_3$) is also used in the making of fertilizer. Baking soda (sodium bicarbonate) is a salt, as are Epsom salts [magnesium sulfate ($MgSO_4$)]. Salt and water can react to form a base and an acid. This is called a **hydrolysis reaction**.

The characteristic properties of acids and bases derive from the tendency of atoms to **ionize** by donating or accepting charged particles. The strength of an acid or base is a reflection of the degree to which its atoms ionize in solution. For example, if all of the atoms in an acid ionize, the acid is said to be **strong**. When only a few of the atoms ionize, the acid is **weak**. Acetic acid ($HC_2H_3O_2$) is a weak acid because only its O_2 atoms ionize in solution. Another way to think of the strength of an acid or base is to consider its **reactivity**. Highly reactive acids and bases are strong because they tend to form and break bonds quickly and most of their atoms ionize in the process.

SI uses the **second** (s) to measure time. Fractions of seconds are usually measured in metric terms using prefixes such as millisecond (1/1,000 of a second) or nanosecond (1/1,000,000,000 of a second). Increments of time larger than a second are measured in minutes and hours, which are multiples of 60 and 24. An example of this is a swimmer's time in the 800-meter freestyle being described as 7:32.67, meaning 7 minutes, 32 seconds, and 67 one-hundredths of a second. One second is equal to 1/60 of a minute, 1/3,600 of an hour, and 1/86,400 of a day.

Other SI base units are the **ampere** (A) (used to measure electric current), the **kelvin** (K) (used to measure thermodynamic temperature), the **candela** (cd) (used to measure luminous intensity), and the **mole** (mol) (used to measure the amount of a substance at a molecular level). **Meter** (m) is used to measure length and **kilogram** (kg) is used to measure mass.

Using the metric system is generally accepted as the preferred method for taking measurements. Having a universal standard allows individuals to interpret measurements more easily, regardless of where they are located.

The basic units of measurement are: the **meter**, which measures length; the **liter**, which measures volume; and the **gram**, which measures mass. The metric system starts with a **base unit** and increases or decreases in units of 10. The prefix and the base unit combined are used to indicate an amount.

For example, deka is 10 times the base unit. A dekameter is 10 meters; a dekaliter is 10 liters; and a dekagram is 10 grams. The prefix hecto refers to 100 times the base amount; kilo is 1,000 times the base amount. The prefixes that indicate a fraction of the base unit are deci, which is 1/10 of the base unit; centi, which is 1/100 of the base unit; and milli, which is 1/1000 of the base unit.

Science – Scientific Reasoning

Describe the prefixes for multiples and subdivisions.

Science – Scientific Reasoning

Describe graduated cylinders and discuss their use.

Science – Scientific Reasoning

Describe the two most commonly used flasks in a lab setting.

Science – Scientific Reasoning

Describe balances and discuss what they measure.

Science – Scientific Reasoning

List the most important considerations when designing an experiment.

Science – Scientific Reasoning

Discuss some key skills necessary to the scientific process: observing, hypothesizing, ordering, categorizing, comparing, inferring, applying, and communicating.

Graduated cylinders are used for an intermediate amount of precision. More precise than beakers and Erlenmeyer flasks but not quite as precise as volumetric flasks or pipettes, they are made of either **polypropylene** (which is shatter-resistant and resistant to chemicals but cannot be heated) or **polymethylpentene** (which is known for its clarity). They are lighter to ship and less fragile than glass.

To read a graduated cylinder, it should be placed on a flat surface and read at eye level. The surface of a liquid in a graduated cylinder forms a lens-shaped curve. The measurement should be taken from the bottom of the curve. A ring may be placed at the top of tall, narrow cylinders to help avoid breakage if they are tipped over.

A **burette**, or buret, is a piece of lab glassware used to accurately dispense liquid. It looks similar to a narrow graduated cylinder, but includes a stopcock and tip. It may be filled with a funnel or pipette.

The prefixes for multiples are as follows:
- deka (da), 10^1 (deka is the American spelling, but deca is also used)
- hecto (h), 10^2
- kilo (k), 10^3
- mega (M), 10^6
- giga (G), 10^9
- tera (T), 10^{12}

The prefixes for subdivisions are as follows:
- deci (d), 10^{-1}
- centi (c), 10^{-2}
- milli (m), 10^{-3}
- micro (μ), 10^{-6}
- nano (n), 10^{-9}
- pico (p), 10^{-12}

The rule of thumb is that prefixes greater than 10^3 are capitalized when abbreviating. Abbreviations do not need a period after them. A decimeter (dm) is a tenth of a meter, a deciliter (dL) is a tenth of a liter, and a decigram (dg) is a tenth of a gram. Pluralization is understood. For example, when referring to 5 mL of water, no "s" needs to be added to the abbreviation.

Unlike laboratory glassware that measures volume, **balances** such as triple-beam balances, spring balances, and electronic balances measure **mass** and **force**. An **electronic balance** is the most accurate, followed by a **triple-beam balance** and then a **spring balance**.

One part of a triple-beam balance is the **plate**, which is where the item to be weighed is placed. There are also three **beams** that have hatch marks indicating amounts and hold the weights that rest in the notches. The front beam measures weights between 0 and 10 grams, the middle beam measures weights in 100-gram increments, and the far beam measures weights in 10-gram increments.

The sum of the weight of each beam is the total weight of the object. A triple-beam balance also includes a **set screw** to calibrate the equipment and a mark indicating the object and counterweights are in balance. Analytical balances are accurate to within 0.0001 g.

Two types of flasks commonly used in lab settings are **Erlenmeyer flasks** and **volumetric flasks**, which can also be used to accurately measure liquids. Erlenmeyer flasks and **beakers** can be used for mixing, transporting, and reacting, but are not appropriate for accurate measurements.

A **pipette** can be used to accurately measure small amounts of liquid. Liquid is drawn into the pipette through the bulb and a finger is then quickly placed at the top of the container. The liquid measurement is read exactly at the **meniscus**. Liquid can be released from the pipette by lifting the finger. There are also plastic disposal pipettes. A **repipette** is a hand-operated pump that dispenses solutions.

Perhaps the most important skill in science is that of **observation**. Scientists must be able to take accurate data from their experimental setup or from nature without allowing bias to alter the results. Another important skill is **hypothesizing**. Scientists must be able to combine their knowledge of theory and of other experimental results to logically determine what should occur in their own tests.

The **data-analysis process** requires the twin skills of ordering and categorizing. Gathered data must be arranged in such a way that it is readable and readily shows the key results. A skill that may be integrated with the previous two is comparing. Scientists should be able to **compare** their own results with other published results. They must also be able to **infer**, or draw logical conclusions, from their results. They must be able to **apply** their knowledge of theory and results to create logical experimental designs and determine cases of special behavior.

Lastly, scientists must be able to **communicate** their results and their conclusions. The greatest scientific progress is made when scientists are able to review and test one another's work and offer advice or suggestions.

A valid experiment must be measurable. **Data tables** should be formed, and meticulous, detailed data should be collected for every trial. First, the researcher must determine exactly what data are needed and why those data are needed. The researcher should know in advance what will be done with those data at the end of the experimental research. The data should be *repeatable, reproducible, and accurate*. The researcher should be sure that the procedure for data collection will be reliable and consistent. The researcher should validate the measurement system by performing **practice tests** and making sure that all of the equipment is correctly **calibrated** and periodically retesting the procedure and equipment to ensure that all data being collected are still valid.

Science – Scientific Reasoning
© Mometrix Media - flashcardsecrets.com/teas
ATI TEAS Exam

Explain some of the different labels given to scientific statements: hypotheses, assumptions, models, laws, and theories.

Science – Scientific Reasoning
© Mometrix Media - flashcardsecrets.com/teas
ATI TEAS Exam

Discuss cause and effect.

Science – Scientific Reasoning
© Mometrix Media - flashcardsecrets.com/teas
ATI TEAS Exam

Discuss how to know which unit of measurement is needed to measure an object.

Science – Scientific Reasoning
© Mometrix Media - flashcardsecrets.com/teas
ATI TEAS Exam

Explain the steps involved in the scientific method of inquiry.

Science – Scientific Reasoning
© Mometrix Media - flashcardsecrets.com/teas
ATI TEAS Exam

Discuss the basics of experimental design.

Science – Scientific Reasoning
© Mometrix Media - flashcardsecrets.com/teas
ATI TEAS Exam

Discuss how to control an experiment.

A **cause** is an act or event that makes something happen, and an **effect** is the thing that happens as a result of the cause. A cause-and-effect relationship is not always explicit, but there are some terms in English that signal causes, such as *since*, *because*, and *due to*. Terms that signal effects include *consequently*, *therefore*, *this lead(s) to*.

A *single* cause can have *multiple* effects (e.g., *Single cause*: Because you left your homework on the table, your dog engulfs the assignment. *Multiple effects*: As a result, you receive a failing grade; your parents do not allow you to visit your friends; you miss out on the new movie and holding the hand of a potential significant other).

A *single* effect can have *multiple* causes (e.g., *Single effect*: Alan has a fever. *Multiple causes*: An unexpected cold front came through the area, and Alan forgot to take his multi-vitamin to avoid being sick.)

An *effect* can in turn be the cause of *another effect*, in what is known as a **cause-and-effect chain**. (e.g., As a result of her disdain for procrastination, Lynn prepared for her exam. This led to her passing her test with high marks. Hence, her resume was accepted and her application was approved.)

Hypotheses are educated guesses about what is likely to occur, and are made to provide a starting point from which to begin design of the experiment. They may be based on results of previously observed experiments or knowledge of theory, and follow logically forth from these.

Assumptions are statements that are taken to be fact without proof for the purpose of performing a given experiment. They may be entirely true, or they may be true only for a given set of conditions under which the experiment will be conducted. Assumptions are necessary to simplify experiments; indeed, many experiments would be impossible without them.

Scientific models are mathematical statements that describe a physical behavior. Models are only as good as our knowledge of the actual system. Often models will be discarded when new discoveries are made that show the model to be inaccurate. While a model can never perfectly represent an actual system, it is useful for simplifying a system to allow for better understanding of its behavior.

Scientific laws are statements of natural behavior that have stood the test of time and have been found to produce accurate and repeatable results in all testing. A **theory** is a statement of behavior that consolidates all current observations. Theories are similar to laws in that they describe natural behavior, but are more recently developed and are more susceptible to being proved wrong. Theories may eventually become laws if they stand up to scrutiny and testing.

The scientific method of inquiry is a general method by which ideas are tested and either confirmed or refuted by experimentation. The first step in the scientific method is **formulating the problem** that is to be addressed. It is essential to define clearly the limits of what is to be observed, since that allows for a more focused analysis.

Once the problem has been defined, it is necessary to form a **hypothesis**. This educated guess should be a possible solution to the problem that was formulated in the first step.

The next step is to test that hypothesis by **experimentation**. This often requires the scientist to design a complete experiment. The key to making the best possible use of an experiment is observation. Observations may be **quantitative**, that is, when a numeric measurement is taken, or they may be **qualitative**, that is, when something is evaluated based on feeling or preference. This measurement data will then be examined to find trends or patterns that are present.

From these trends, the scientist will draw **conclusions** or make **generalizations** about the results, intended to predict future results. If these conclusions support the original hypothesis, the experiment is complete and the scientist will publish his conclusions to allow others to test them by repeating the experiment. If they do not support the hypothesis, the results should then be used to develop a new hypothesis, which can then be verified by a new or redesigned experiment.

From the largest objects in outer space to the smallest pieces of the human body, there are objects that can come in many different sizes and shapes. Many of those objects need to be measured in different ways. So, it is important to know which **unit of measurement** is needed to record the length or width and the weight of an object.

An example is taking the measurements of a patient. When measuring the total height of a patient or finding the length of an extremity, the accepted measure is given in meters. However, when one is asked for the diameter of a vein, the accepted measure is given in millimeters. Another example would be measuring the weight of a patient which would be given in kilograms, while the measurement of a human heart would be given in grams. The same idea for scale holds true with time as well. When measuring the lifespan of a patient, the accepted measure is given in days, months, or years. However, when measuring the number of breaths that a patient takes, the accepted measure is given in terms of minutes (e.g., breaths per minute).

A valid experiment must be carefully **controlled**. All variables except the one being tested must be carefully maintained. This means that all conditions must be kept exactly the same except for the independent variable.

Additionally, a set of data is usually needed for a **control group**. The control group represents the "normal" state or condition of the variable being manipulated. Controls can be negative or positive. **Positive controls** are the variables that the researcher expects to have an effect on the outcome of the experiment. A positive control group can be used to verify that an experiment is set up properly. **Negative control groups** are typically thought of as placebos. A negative control group should verify that a variable has no effect on the outcome of the experiment.

The better an experiment is controlled, the more valid the conclusions from that experiment will be. A researcher is more likely to draw a valid conclusion if all variables other than the one being manipulated are being controlled.

Designing relevant experiments that allow for meaningful results is not a simple task. Every stage of the experiment must be carefully planned to ensure that the right data can be safely and accurately taken.

Ideally, an experiment should be **controlled** so that all of the conditions except the ones being manipulated are held **constant**. This helps to ensure that the results are not skewed by unintended consequences of shifting conditions. A good example of this is a placebo group in a drug trial. All other conditions are the same, but that group is not given the medication.

In addition to proper control, it is important that the experiment be designed with **data collection** in mind. For instance, if the quantity to be measured is temperature, there must be a temperature device such as a thermocouple integrated into the experimental setup. While the data are being collected, they should periodically be checked for obvious errors. If there are data points that are orders of magnitude from the expected value, then it might be a good idea to make sure that no experimental errors are being made, either in data collection or condition control.

Once all the data have been gathered, they must be **analyzed**. The way in which this should be done depends on the type of data and the type of trends observed. It may be useful to fit curves to the data to determine if the trends follow a common mathematical form. It may also be necessary to perform a statistical analysis of the results to determine what effects are significant. Data should be clearly presented.

Science – Scientific Reasoning
© Mometrix Media - flashcardsecrets.com/teas
ATI TEAS Exam

Discuss variables within an experiment.

Visit *mometrix.com/academy* for related videos.
Enter video codes: 627181 and 565738

English and Language Usage - Conventions of Standard English
© Mometrix Media - flashcardsecrets.com/teas
ATI TEAS Exam

State the spelling rules for words ending with a consonant.

English and Language Usage - Conventions of Standard English
© Mometrix Media - flashcardsecrets.com/teas
ATI TEAS Exam

Name the spelling rules for words ending in *y* or *c*.

English and Language Usage - Conventions of Standard English
© Mometrix Media - flashcardsecrets.com/teas
ATI TEAS Exam

Name the spelling rules for words ending in *ie*, *ei*, or *e*.

English and Language Usage - Conventions of Standard English
© Mometrix Media - flashcardsecrets.com/teas
ATI TEAS Exam

State the spelling rules for words ending with *is*, or *ize*.

English and Language Usage - Conventions of Standard English
© Mometrix Media - flashcardsecrets.com/teas
ATI TEAS Exam

State the spelling rules for words ending with *ceed*, *sede*, or *cede*.

Usually the final consonant is **doubled** on a word before adding a suffix. This is the rule for single syllable words, words ending with one consonant, and multi-syllable words with the last syllable accented. The following are examples:
- *beg* becomes *begging* (single syllable)
- *shop* becomes *shopped* (single syllable)
- *add* becomes *adding* (already ends in double consonant, do not add another *d*)
- *deter* becomes *deterring* (multi-syllable, accent on last syllable)
- *regret* becomes *regrettable* (multi-syllable, accent on last syllable)
- *compost* becomes *composting* (do not add another *t* because the accent is on the first syllable)

Every experiment has several **variables**; however, only one variable should be purposely changed and tested. This variable is the **manipulated** or **independent variable**. As this variable is manipulated or changed, another variable, called the **responding** or **dependent variable**, is observed and recorded.

All other variables in the experiment must be carefully controlled and are usually referred to as **constants**. For example, when testing the effect of temperature on solubility of a solute, the independent variable is the temperature, and the dependent variable is the solubility. All other factors in the experiment such as pressure, amount of stirring, type of solvent, type of solute, and particle size of the solute are the constants.

Most words are spelled with an *i* before *e*, except when they follow the letter *c*, or sound like *a*. For example, the following words are spelled correctly according to these rules:
- piece, friend, believe (*i* before *e*)
- receive, ceiling, conceited (except after *c*)
- weight, neighborhood, veil (sounds like *a*)

To add a suffix to words ending with the letter *e*, first determine if the *e* is silent. If it is, the *e* will be kept if the added suffix begins with a consonant. If the suffix begins with a vowel, the *e* is dropped. The following are examples:
- *age* becomes *ageless* (keep the *e*)
- *age* becomes *aging* (drop the *e*)

An exception to this rule occurs when the word ends in *ce* or *ge* and the suffix *able* or *ous* is added; these words will retain the letter *e*. The following are examples:
- courage becomes courageous
- notice becomes noticeable

The general rule for words ending in *y* is to keep the *y* when adding a suffix if the **y is preceded by a vowel**. If the word **ends in a consonant and y** the *y* is changed to an *i* before the suffix is added (unless the suffix itself begins with *i*). The following are examples:
- *pay* becomes *paying* (keep the *y*)
- *bully* becomes *bullied* (change to *i*)
- *bully* becomes *bullying* (keep the *y* because the suffix is –*ing*)

If a word ends with *c* and the suffix begins with an *e*, *i*, or *y*, the letter *k* is usually added to the end of the word. The following are examples:
- panic becomes panicky
- mimic becomes mimicking

There are only three words in the English language that end with *ceed*: *exceed, proceed,* and *succeed*. There is only one word in the English language that ends with *sede*: *supersede*. Most other words that sound like *sede* or *ceed* end with *cede*. The following are examples:
- concede, recede, and precede

A small number of words end with *ise*. Most of the words in the English language with the same sound end in *ize*. The following are examples:
- advertise, advise, arise, chastise, circumcise, and comprise
- compromise, demise, despise, devise, disguise, enterprise, excise, and exercise
- franchise, improvise, incise, merchandise, premise, reprise, and revise
- supervise, surmise, surprise, and televise

Words that end with *ize* include the following:
- accessorize, agonize, authorize, and brutalize
- capitalize, caramelize, categorize, civilize, and demonize
- downsize, empathize, euthanize, idolize, and immunize
- legalize, metabolize, mobilize, organize, and ostracize
- plagiarize, privatize, utilize, and visualize

(Note that some words may technically be spelled with *ise*, especially in British English, but it is more common to use *ize*. Examples include *symbolize/symbolise* and *baptize/baptise*.)

State the rules for words ending in *able* or *ible*.

Discuss the rules for words ending in *ance* or *ence*.

State the spelling rules for words ending *tion, sion,* or *cian*.

State the rules for words with the *ai* or *ia* combination.

Discuss the plural forms of nouns ending in ch, sh, s, x, or z.

Discuss the plural forms of nouns ending in *y* or *ay / ey / iy / oy / uy*.

The suffixes *ence, ency,* and *ent* are used in the following cases:
- the suffix is preceded by the letter *c* but sounds like *s* – *innocence*
- the suffix is preceded by the letter *g* but sounds like *j* – *intelligence, negligence*

The suffixes *ance, ancy,* and *ant* are used in the following cases:
- the suffix is preceded by the letter *c* but sounds like *k* – *significant, vacant*
- the suffix is preceded by the letter *g* with a hard sound – *elegant, extravagance*

If the suffix is preceded by other letters, there are no clear rules. For example: *finance, abundance,* and *assistance* use the letter *a,* while *decadence, competence,* and *excellence* use the letter *e.*

For words ending in *able* or *ible*, there are no hard and fast rules. The following are examples:
- adjustable, unbeatable, collectable, deliverable, and likeable
- edible, compatible, feasible, sensible, and credible

There are more words ending in *able* than *ible*; this is useful to know if guessing is necessary.

When deciding if *ai* or *ia* is correct, the combination of *ai* usually sounds like one vowel sound, as in *Britain*, while the vowels in *ia* are pronounced separately, as in *guardian*. The following are examples:
- captain, certain, faint, hair, malaise, and praise (*ai* makes one sound)
- bacteria, beneficiary, diamond, humiliation, and nuptial (*ia* makes two sounds)

Words ending in *tion, sion,* or *cian* all sound like *shun* or *zhun*. There are no rules for which ending is used for words. The following are examples:
- action, agitation, caution, fiction, nation, and motion
- admission, expression, mansion, permission, and television
- electrician, magician, musician, optician, and physician (note that these words tend to describe occupations)

If a noun ends with a **consonant and y**, the plural is formed by replacing the *y* with *ies*. For example, *fly* becomes *flies* and *puppy* becomes *puppies*. If a noun ends with a **vowel and y**, the plural is formed by adding an *s*. For example, *alley* becomes *alleys* and *boy* becomes *boys*.

When a noun ends in the letters *ch, sh, s, x,* or *z*, an *es* instead of a singular *s* is added to the end of the word to make it plural. The following are examples:
- church becomes churches
- bush becomes bushes
- bass becomes basses
- mix becomes mixes
- buzz becomes buzzes

This is the rule with proper names as well; the Ross family would become the Rosses.

Discuss the plural forms of nouns ending in *f* or *fe*.

Discuss the plural forms of nouns ending in *o*.

Explain some exceptions to the rules of plurals.

Discuss the plural forms of letters, numbers, symbols, and compound nouns with hyphens.

Define and discuss homophones.

Differentiate between the following frequently confused words:
    affect and effect
    its and it's

Most nouns ending with a **consonant and *o*** are pluralized by adding *es*. The following are examples:
- hero becomes heroes; tornado becomes tornadoes; potato becomes potatoes

Most nouns ending with a **vowel and *o*** are pluralized by adding *s*. The following are examples:
- portfolio becomes portfolios; radio becomes radios; cameo becomes cameos.

An exception to these rules is seen with musical terms ending in *o*. These words are pluralized by adding *s* even if they end in a consonant and *o*. The following are examples: *soprano* becomes *sopranos*; *banjo* becomes *banjos*; *piano* becomes *pianos*.

Most nouns ending in *f* or *fe* are pluralized by replacing the *f* with *v* and adding *es*. The following are examples:
- knife becomes knives; self becomes selves; wolf becomes wolves.
- An exception to this rule is the word *roof*; *roof* becomes *roofs*.

Letters and numbers become plural by adding an apostrophe and *s*. The following are examples:
- The *L's* are the people whose names begin with the letter *L*.
- They broke the teams down into groups of *3's*.
- The sorority girls were all *KD's*.

A **compound noun** is a noun that is made up of two or more words; they can be written with hyphens. For example, *mother-in-law* or *court-martial* are compound nouns. To make them plural, an *s* or *es* is added to the noun portion of the word. The following are examples: *mother-in-law* becomes *mothers-in-law*; *court-martial* becomes *courts-martial*.

Some words do not fall into any specific category for making the singular form plural. They are **irregular**. Certain words become plural by changing the vowels within the word. The following are examples:
- woman becomes women; goose becomes geese; foot becomes feet

Some words change in unusual ways in the plural form. The following are examples:
- mouse becomes mice; ox becomes oxen; person becomes people

Some words are the same in both the singular and plural forms. The following are examples:
- *Salmon*, *deer*, and *moose* are the same whether singular or plural.

Affect can be used as a noun for feeling, emotion, or mood. Effect can be used as a noun that means result. Affect as a verb means to influence. Effect as a verb means to bring about.

Affect: The sunshine affects plants.
Effect: The new rules will effect order in the office.

Its and It's
Its is a pronoun that shows ownership.

Example: The guitar is in its case.

It's is a contraction of *it is*.

Example: It's an honor and a privilege to meet you.

Note: The *h* in honor is silent. So, the sound of the vowel *o* must have the article *an*.

Homophones are words that are **pronounced** in the same way, but they have different **spellings** and different **meanings**. It's easy to make a mistake and use the wrong word when writing. So, it's important to make sure you choose the correct word.
Examples

bare, bear	for, four	knot, not	plain, plane	stair, stare
brake, break	heal, heel	know, no	pour, poor	steal, steel
buy, by	hear, here	mail, male	principal, principle	toe, tow
dear, deer	hole, whole	pair, pear	right, write	wait, weight
flour, flower	hour, our	peace, piece	son, sun	waist, waste

English and Language Usage - Conventions of Standard English
© Mometrix Media - flashcardsecrets.com/teas
ATI TEAS Exam

Differentiate between the following frequently confused words:
  knew and new
  there, their, and they're

English and Language Usage - Conventions of Standard English
© Mometrix Media - flashcardsecrets.com/teas
ATI TEAS Exam

Differentiate between the following frequently confused words:
  to, too, and two
  your and you're

English and Language Usage - Conventions of Standard English
© Mometrix Media - flashcardsecrets.com/teas
ATI TEAS Exam

Define and discuss homographs.

English and Language Usage - Conventions of Standard English
© Mometrix Media - flashcardsecrets.com/teas
ATI TEAS Exam

Give at least two meanings for each of the following homographs:
  bank
  content
  fine
  incense

English and Language Usage - Conventions of Standard English
© Mometrix Media - flashcardsecrets.com/teas
ATI TEAS Exam

Give at least two meanings for each of the following homographs:
  lead
  object
  produce
  refuse

English and Language Usage - Conventions of Standard English
© Mometrix Media - flashcardsecrets.com/teas
ATI TEAS Exam

Give at least two meanings for each of the following homographs:
  subject
  tear

To, Too, and Two
To can be an adverb or a preposition for showing direction, purpose, and relationship. See your dictionary for the many other ways use *to* in a sentence.
Examples: I went to the store. | I want to go with you.

Too is an adverb that means *also, as well, very, or more than enough*.
Examples: I can walk a mile too. | You have eaten too much.

Two is the second number in the series of natural numbers (e.g., one (1), two, (2), three (3)…)
Example: You have two minutes left.

Your and You're
Your is an adjective that shows ownership.
Example: This is your moment to shine.

You're is a contraction of you are.
Example: Yes, you're correct.

Knew and New
Knew is the past tense of *know*.
Example: I knew the answer.

New is an adjective that means something is current, has not been used, or modern.
Example: This is my new phone.

There, Their, and They're
There can be an adjective, adverb, or pronoun. Often, *there* is used to show a place or to start a sentence.
Examples: I went there yesterday. | There is something in his pocket.

Their is a pronoun that shows ownership.
Examples: He is their father. | This is their fourth apology this week.

They're is a contraction of *they are*.
Example: Did you know that they're in town?

Bank
(noun): an establishment where money is held for savings or lending
(verb): to collect or pile up

Content
(noun): the topics that will be addressed within a book
(adjective): pleased or satisfied

Fine
(noun): an amount of money that acts a penalty for an offense
(adjective): very small or thin

Incense
(noun): a material that is burned in religious settings and makes a pleasant aroma
(verb): to frustrate or anger

Homographs are words that share the same **spelling**, and they have multiple meanings. To figure out which meaning is being used, you should be looking for **context clues**. The context clues give hints to the meaning of the word. For example, the word *spot* has many meanings. It can mean "a place" or "a stain or blot." In the sentence "After my lunch, I saw a spot on my shirt," the word *spot* means "a stain or blot." The context clues of "After my lunch…" and "on my shirt" guide you to this decision.

Subject
(noun): an area of study
(verb): to force or subdue

Tear
(noun): a fluid secreted by the eyes
(verb): to separate or pull apart

Lead
(noun): the first or highest position
(verb): to direct a person or group of followers

Object
(noun): a lifeless item that can be held and observed
(verb): to disagree

Produce
(noun): fruits and vegetables
(verb): to make or create something

Refuse
(noun): garbage or debris that has been thrown away
(verb): to not allow

Define common nouns and proper nouns.

Define general nouns, specific nouns, and collective nouns.

Describe pronouns and their uses.

Discuss how pronouns can be grouped.

Visit *mometrix.com/academy* for a related video.
Enter video code: 312073

Describe transitive and intransitive verbs and discuss their uses.

Describe action verbs and linking verbs.

When you talk about a person, place, thing, or idea, you are talking about **nouns**. The two main types of nouns are common and proper nouns. Also, nouns can be abstract (i.e., general) or concrete (i.e., specific).

Common nouns are the class or group of people, places, and things (Note: do not capitalize common nouns). Examples of common nouns:
People: boy, girl, worker, manager
Places: school, bank, library, home
Things: dog, cat, truck, car

Proper nouns are the names of specific persons, places, or things (Note: capitalize all proper nouns). Examples of proper nouns:
People: Abraham Lincoln, George Washington, Martin Luther King, Jr.
Places: Los Angeles, New York, Asia
Things: Statue of Liberty, Earth*, Lincoln Memorial
*Note: When you talk about the planet that we live on, you capitalize *Earth*. When you mean the dirt, rocks, or land, you lowercase *earth*.

General nouns are the names of conditions or ideas. **Specific nouns** name people, places, and things that are understood by using your senses.

General nouns:
Condition: beauty, strength
Idea: truth, peace

Specific nouns:
People: baby, friend, father
Places: town, park, city hall
Things: rainbow, cough, apple, silk, gasoline

Collective nouns are the names for a person, place, or thing that may act as a whole. The following are examples of collective nouns: *class, company, dozen, group, herd, team,* and *public*.

Pronouns are words that are used to stand in for a noun. A pronoun may be grouped as *personal, intensive, relative, interrogative, demonstrative, indefinite,* and *reciprocal*.

Personal: Nominative is the case for nouns and pronouns that are the subject of a sentence. **Objective** is the case for nouns and pronouns that are an object in a sentence. **Possessive** is the case for nouns and pronouns that show possession or ownership.

Singular

	Nominative	Objective	Possessive
First Person	I	me	my, mine
Second Person	you	you	your, yours
Third Person	he, she, it	him, her, it	his, her, hers, its

Plural

	Nominative	Objective	Possessive
First Person	we	us	our, ours
Second Person	you	you	your, yours
Third Person	they	them	their, theirs

Intensive: I myself, you yourself, he himself, she herself, the (thing) itself, we ourselves, you yourselves, they themselves

Relative: which, who, whom, whose

Interrogative: what, which, who, whom, whose

Demonstrative: this, that, these, those

Indefinite: all, any, each, everyone, either/neither, one, some, several

Reciprocal: each other, one another

If you want to write a sentence, then you need a **verb** in your sentence. Without a verb, you have no sentence. The verb of a sentence explains **action** or **being**. In other words, the verb shows the subject's movement or the movement that has been done to the subject.

Transitive and Intransitive Verbs
A **transitive verb** is a verb whose action (e.g., drive, run, jump) points to a receiver (e.g., car, dog, kangaroo). **Intransitive verbs** do not point to a receiver of an action. In other words, the action of the verb does not point to a subject or object.

Transitive: He plays the piano. | The piano was played by him.

Intransitive: He plays. | John writes well.

A dictionary will let you know whether a verb is transitive or intransitive. Some verbs can be transitive and intransitive.

An action verb is a verb that shows what the subject is doing in a sentence. In other words, an **action verb** shows action. A sentence can be complete with one word: an action verb. **Linking verbs** are intransitive verbs that show a condition (i.e., the subject is described but does no action).

Linking verbs link the **subject** of a sentence to a **noun or pronoun**, or they link a subject with an **adjective**. You always need a verb if you want a complete sentence. However, linking verbs are not able to complete a sentence.

Common linking verbs include *appear, be, become, feel, grow, look, seem, smell, sound,* and *taste*. However, any verb that shows a condition and has a noun, pronoun, or adjective that describes the subject of a sentence is a linking verb.

Action: He sings. | Run! | Go! | I talk with him every day. | She reads.
Linking: I am John. | I smell roses. | I feel tired.

Note: Some verbs are followed by words that look like prepositions, but they are a part of the verb and a part of the verb's meaning. These are known as **phrasal verbs** and examples include *call off, look up,* and *drop off*.

Discuss transitive verbs with active and passive voice.

Discuss verb tenses.

Discuss perfect verb tenses.

Describe the process of conjugating verbs.

Visit *mometrix.com/academy* for a related video.
Enter video code: 269472

Discuss indicative, imperative, and subjunctive moods.

Define adjectives and discuss their function.

A verb tense shows the different form of a verb to point to the time of an action. The **present** and **past tense** are shown by changing the verb's form. An action in the present *I talk* can change form for the past: *I talked*. However, for the other tenses, an **auxiliary** (i.e., helping) verb is needed to show the change in form. These helping verbs include *am, are, is | have, has, had | was, were, will* (or *shall*).

Present: I talk	Present perfect: I have talked
Past: I talked	Past perfect: I had talked
Future: I will talk	Future perfect: I will have talked

Present: The action happens at the current time.
Example: He *walks* to the store every morning.
To show that something is happening right now, use the progressive present tense: I *am walking*.

Past: The action happened in the past.
Example: He *walked* to the store an hour ago.

Future: The action is going to happen later.
Example: I *will walk* to the store tomorrow.

When you need to change the form of a verb, you are **conjugating** a verb. The key parts of a verb are **first person singular**, **present tense** (dream); **first person singular**, **past tense** (dreamed); and the **past participle** (dreamed). Note: the past participle needs a helping verb to make a verb tense. For example, I *have dreamed* of this day. | I *am dreaming* of this day.

Present Tense: Active Voice

	Singular	Plural
First Person	I dream	We dream
Second Person	You dream	You dream
Third Person	He, she, it dreams	They dream

An adjective is a word that is used to **modify** a noun or pronoun. An adjective answers a question: *Which one?*, *What kind of?*, or *How many?*. Usually, adjectives come before the words that they modify.

Which one: The *third* suit is my favorite.
How many: Can I look over the *four* neckties for the suit?

Transitive verbs come in active or passive voice. If the subject does an action or receives the action of the verb, then you will know whether a verb is active or passive. When the subject of the sentence is doing the action, the verb is **active voice**. When the subject receives the action, the verb is **passive voice**.

Active: Jon drew the picture. (The subject *Jon* is doing the action of *drawing a picture*.)

Passive: The picture is drawn by Jon. (The subject *picture* is receiving the action from Jon.)

Present perfect: The action started in the past and continues into the present.
Example: I *have walked* to the store three times today.

Past perfect: The second action happened in the past. The first action came before the second.
Example: Before I walked to the store (Action 2), I *had walked* to the library (Action 1).

Future perfect: An action that uses the past and the future. In other words, the action is complete before a future moment.
Example: When she comes for the supplies (future moment), I *will have walked* to the store (action completed in the past).

There are three moods in English: the indicative, the imperative, and the subjunctive.

The **indicative mood** is used for facts, opinions, and questions.
Fact: You can do this.
Opinion: I think that you can do this.
Question: Do you know that you can do this?

The **imperative** is used for orders or requests.
Order: You are going to do this!
Request: Will you do this for me?

The **subjunctive mood** is for wishes and statements that go against fact.
Wish: I wish that I were going to do this.
Statement against fact: If I were you, I would do this. (This goes against fact because I am not you. You have the chance to do this, and I do not have the chance.)

The mood that causes trouble for most people is the subjunctive mood. If you have trouble with any of the moods, then be sure to practice.

English and Language Usage - Conventions of Standard English
© Mometrix Media - flashcardsecrets.com/teas
ATI TEAS Exam

Define and discuss articles.

English and Language Usage - Conventions of Standard English
© Mometrix Media - flashcardsecrets.com/teas
ATI TEAS Exam

Describe relative and absolute adjectives.

Visit *mometrix.com/academy* for a related video.
Enter video code: 470154

English and Language Usage - Conventions of Standard English
© Mometrix Media - flashcardsecrets.com/teas
ATI TEAS Exam

Define and discuss adverbs.

English and Language Usage - Conventions of Standard English
© Mometrix Media - flashcardsecrets.com/teas
ATI TEAS Exam

Describe the rules for comparing adverbs and adjectives.

Visit *mometrix.com/academy* for a related video.
Enter video code: 400865

English and Language Usage - Conventions of Standard English
© Mometrix Media - flashcardsecrets.com/teas
ATI TEAS Exam

Define, in depth, prepositions and how they are used.

Visit *mometrix.com/academy* for a related video.
Enter video code: 946763

English and Language Usage - Conventions of Standard English
© Mometrix Media - flashcardsecrets.com/teas
ATI TEAS Exam

Define, in depth, conjunctions and how they are used.

Visit *mometrix.com/academy* for a related video.
Enter video code: 390329

Some adjectives are relative and other adjectives are absolute. Adjectives that are **relative** can show the comparison between things. Adjectives that are **absolute** can show comparison. However, they show comparison in a different way. Let's say that you are reading two books. You think that one book is perfect, and the other book is not exactly perfect. It is <u>not</u> possible for the book to be more perfect than the other. Either you think that the book is perfect, or you think that the book is not perfect.

The adjectives that are relative will show the different **degrees** of something or someone to something else or someone else. The three degrees of adjectives include positive, comparative, and superlative.

The **positive degree** is the normal form of an adjective.
Example: This work is *difficult*. | She is *smart*.

The **comparative degree** compares one person or thing to another person or thing.
Example: This work is *more difficult* than your work. | She is *smarter* than me.

The **superlative degree** compares more than two people or things.
Example: This is the *most difficult* work of my life. | She is the *smartest* lady in school.

Articles are adjectives that are used to **mark nouns**. There are only three: the definite (i.e., limited or fixed amount) article *the*, and the indefinite (i.e., no limit or fixed amount) articles *a* and *an*. Note: *An* comes before words that start with a vowel sound (i.e., vowels include *a, e, i, o, u,* and *y*). For example, Are you going to get an **u**mbrella?

Definite: I lost *the* bottle that belongs to me.
Indefinite: Does anyone have *a* bottle to share?

The rules for comparing adverbs are the same as the rules for adjectives.

The **positive degree** is the standard form of an adverb.
Example: He arrives soon. | She speaks softly to her friends.

The **comparative degree** compares one person or thing to another person or thing.
Example: He arrives sooner than Sarah. | She speaks more softly than him.

The **superlative degree** compares more than two people or things.
Example: He arrives soonest of the group. | She speaks most softly of any of her friends.

An adverb is a word that is used to **modify** a verb, adjective, or another adverb. Usually, adverbs answer one of these questions: *When?, Where?, How?,* and *Why?* . The negatives *not* and *never* are known as adverbs. Adverbs that modify adjectives or other adverbs strengthen or weaken the words that they modify.

Examples:
He walks quickly through the crowd.
The water flows smoothly on the rocks.

Note: While many adverbs end in *-ly*, you need to remember that not all adverbs end in *-ly*. Also, some words that end in *-ly* are adjectives, not adverbs. Some examples include: *early, friendly, holy, lonely, silly,* and *ugly*. To know if a word that ends in *-ly* is an adjective or adverb, you can check whether it answers one of the adjective questions or one of the adverb questions.

Examples:
He is *never* angry.
You talk *too* loudly.

Conjunctions **join** words, phrases, or clauses, and they show the connection between the joined pieces. There are **coordinating conjunctions** that connect equal parts of sentences. **Correlative conjunctions** show the connection between pairs. **Subordinating conjunctions** join subordinate (i.e., dependent) clauses with independent clauses.

Coordinating Conjunctions
The coordinating conjunctions include: *and, but, yet, or, nor, for,* and *so*
Examples:
The rock was small, but it was heavy.
She drove in the night, and he drove in the day.

Correlative Conjunctions
The correlative conjunctions are: either...or | neither...nor | not only... but also
Examples:
Either you are coming, or you are staying.
He not only ran three miles, but also swam 200 yards.

A preposition is a word placed before a noun or pronoun that shows the *relationship between an object and another word* in the sentence.

Common Prepositions:

about	before	during	on	under
after	beneath	for	over	until
against	between	from	past	up
among	beyond	in	through	with
around	by	of	to	within
at	down	off	toward	without

Examples:
The napkin is *in* the drawer.
The Earth rotates *around* the Sun.
The needle is *beneath* the haystack.
Can you find me *among* the words?

English and Language Usage - Conventions of Standard English

Discuss common subordinating conjunctions.

Visit *mometrix.com/academy* for a related video.
Enter video code: 958913

English and Language Usage - Conventions of Standard English

Define and discuss interjections.

English and Language Usage - Conventions of Standard English

Provide the correct spelling for any misspelled words:

accidentaly	existance	occurrence
achieved	explaination	omited
aparently	Febuary	operate
calender	finally	optamistic
changeing	hopeing	parallel
chauffeur	iminent	physicaly
colonel	inocence	possess
concieve	library	predjudice
defered	litrature	psycholgy
desireable	matress	recede
disapoint	mortgage	schedule
dissatisfied	neice	sophmore
exaggerate	occasion	tournement

English and Language Usage - Conventions of Standard English

Provide the correct spelling for any misspelled words:

acknowledgment	disese	rhetiric
accross	drudgry	salary
aisle	extasy	scarcely
artic	eighth	secratary
arangement	independant	sherrif
awkward	iresistible	sufrage
bachlor	liable	supress
biscuit	obsticle	temprament
cafeteria	persuade	temprature
cemetary	practicaly	tendancy
desparate	prarie	unanimous
diptheria	religious	valueable
discapline	restaurant	wholely

English and Language Usage - Conventions of Standard English

Provide the correct spelling for any misspelled words:

accomodate	discusion	ninety
adress	eligable	notoriaty
aggravate	emphasise	pagent
apearance	forehead	permissable
beneficary	foreign	prevelent
candidate	glamorus	rally
changable	government	referal
compell	hypocrisey	rhythm
consious	incredible	severly
coolly	judgement	transfered
deceive	legitamate	vengence
deferance	momentus	weird
describe	nickle	yolk

English and Language Usage - Conventions of Standard English

Provide the correct spelling for any misspelled words:

barbarian	greivous	Referred
committ	hankerchief	resistence
commitee	hygeine	ridiculus
competition	intentionaly	sacreligious
conqurer	manual	sentinal
disastrius	mathmatics	shriek
especially	organisation	species
exhaust	outrageus	studying
familar	parlament	supercede
formost	preceeding	symetry
ghost	pronunciation	twelvth
glamorus	propeler	useage
grief	recomend	Wednesday

An interjection is a word for **exclamation** (i.e., great amount of feeling) that is used alone or as a piece to a sentence. Often, they are used at the beginning of a sentence for an **introduction**. Sometimes, they can be used in the middle of a sentence to show a **change** in thought or attitude.

Common Interjections: Hey! | Oh, ... | Ouch! | Please! | Wow!

Common subordinating conjunctions include:

after	since	whenever
although	so that	where
because	unless	wherever
before	until	whether
in order that	when	while

Examples:
I am hungry *because* I did not eat breakfast.
He went home *when* everyone left.

Spelling words

INCORRECT	CORRECT	INCORRECT	CORRECT
	acknowledgment	obsticle	obstacle
accross	across		persuade
	aisle	practicaly	practically
artic	arctic	prarie	prairie
arangement	arrangement		religious
	awkward		restaurant
bachlor	bachelor	rhetiric	rhetoric
	biscuit		salary
	cafeteria		scarcely
cemetary	cemetery	secratary	secretary
desparate	desperate	sherrif	sheriff
diptheria	diphtheria	sufrage	suffrage
discapline	discipline	supress	suppress
disese	disease	temprament	temperament
drudgry	drudgery	temprature	temperature
extasy	ecstasy	tendancy	tendency
	eighth		unanimous
independant	independent	valueable	valuable
iresistible	irresistible	wholely	wholly
	liable		

Spelling words

INCORRECT	CORRECT	INCORRECT	CORRECT
accidentaly	accidentally	inocence	innocence
	achieved		library
aparently	apparently	litrature	literature
calender	calendar	matress	mattress
changeing	changing		mortgage
	chauffeur	neice	niece
	colonel		occasion
concieve	conceive		occurrence
defered	deferred	omited	omitted
desireable	desirable		operate
disapoint	disappoint	optamistic	optimistic
	dissatisfied		parallel
	exaggerate	physicaly	physically
existance	existence		possess
explaination	explanation	predjudice	prejudice
Febuary	February	psycholgy	psychology
	finally		recede
hopeing	hoping		schedule
iminent	imminent	sophmore	sophomore
		tournement	tournament

Spelling words

INCORRECT	CORRECT	INCORRECT	CORRECT
	barbarian	outrageus	outrageous
committ	commit	parlament	parliament
commitee	committee	preceeding	preceding
	competition		pronunciation
conqurer	conqueror	propeler	propeller
disastrius	disastrous	recomend	recommend
	especially	refered	referred
	exhaust	resistence	resistance
familar	familiar	ridiculus	ridiculous
formost	foremost	sacreligious	sacrilegious
	ghost	sentinal	sentinel
glamorus	glamorous		shriek
	grief		species
greivous	grievous		studying
hankerchief	handkerchief	supercede	supersede
hygeine	hygiene	symetry	symmetry
intentionaly	intentionally	twelvth	twelfth
	manual	useage	usage
mathmatics	mathematics		Wednesday
organisation	organization		

Spelling words

INCORRECT	CORRECT	INCORRECT	CORRECT
accomodate	accommodate	hypocrisey	hypocrisy
adress	address		incredible
	aggravate	judgement	judgment
apearance	appearance	legitamate	legitimate
beneficary	beneficiary	momentus	momentous
	candidate	nickle	nickel
changable	changeable		ninety
compell	compel	notoriaty	notoriety
consious	conscious	pagent	pageant
	coolly	permissable	permissible
	deceive	prevelent	prevalent
deferance	deference		rally
	describe	referal	referral
discusion	discussion		rhythm
eligable	eligible	severly	severely
emphasise	emphasize	transfered	transferred
	forehead	vengence	vengeance
	foreign		weird
glamorus	glamorous		yolk
	government		

English and Language Usage - Punctuation
ATI TEAS Exam

Discuss declarative and imperative sentences.

English and Language Usage - Punctuation
ATI TEAS Exam

Discuss the use of question marks, exclamation marks, and periods for abbreviations.

English and Language Usage - Punctuation
ATI TEAS Exam

Describe the use of commas in general and in the following situations:
- before a coordinating conjunction
- after an introductory phrase
- between items in a series

Visit *mometrix.com/academy* for a related video.
Enter video code: 786797

English and Language Usage - Punctuation
ATI TEAS Exam

Describe the use of commas in the following situations:
- between coordinate adjectives
- after interjections and yes/no
- separating nonessential phrases

English and Language Usage - Punctuation
ATI TEAS Exam

Describe the use of commas in the following situations:
- direct address, interrogative tags, and contrasts
- dates, address, geographical names, and titles
- *he/she said* in the middle of a quotation

English and Language Usage - Punctuation
ATI TEAS Exam

Describe the use of semicolons.

Visit *mometrix.com/academy* for a related video.
Enter video code: 370605

Question Marks
Question marks should be used following a direct question. A polite request can be followed by a period instead of a question mark.
Direct Question: What is for lunch today? | How are you? | Why is that the answer?
Polite Requests: Can you please send me the item tomorrow. | Will you please walk with me.

Exclamation Marks
Exclamation marks are used after a word group or sentence that shows much feeling or has special importance. Exclamation marks should not be overused. They are saved for proper **exclamatory interjections**.
Examples: We're going to the finals! | You have a beautiful car! | That's crazy!

Special Note
Periods for Abbreviations
An abbreviation is a shortened form of a word or phrase.
Examples: 3 P.M. | 2 A.M. | Mr. Jones | Mrs. Stevens | Dr. Smith | Bill Jr. | Pennsylvania Ave.

Use a period to end all sentences except direct questions, exclamations, and questions.

Declarative Sentence
A declarative sentence gives information or makes a statement.
Examples: I can fly a kite. | The plane left two hours ago.

Imperative Sentence
An imperative sentence gives an order or command.
Examples: You are coming with me. | Bring me that note.

Use a comma between **coordinate adjectives** not joined with *and*
Incorrect: The kind, brown dog followed me home.
Correct: The *kind, loyal* dog followed me home.

Not all adjectives are coordinate (i.e., equal or parallel). There are two simple ways to know if your adjectives are coordinate. One, you can join the adjectives with *and*: *The kind and loyal dog*. Two, you can change the order of the adjectives: *The loyal, kind dog*.

Use commas for **interjections** and **after** *yes* and *no* **responses**
Examples:
Interjection: Oh, I had no idea. | Wow, you know how to play this game.
Yes and No: *Yes,* I heard you. | *No,* I cannot come tomorrow.

Use commas to **separate nonessential modifiers** and **nonessential appositives**
Examples:
Nonessential Modifier: John Frank, who is coaching the team, was promoted today.
Nonessential Appositive: Thomas Edison, an American inventor, was born in Ohio.

The comma is a punctuation mark that can help you understand **connections** in a sentence. Not every sentence needs a comma. However, if a sentence needs a comma, you need to put it in the right place. A comma in the wrong place (or an absent comma) will make a sentence's meaning unclear. These are some of the rules for commas:

Use a comma before a **coordinating conjunction** joining independent clauses
Example: *Bob caught three fish, and I caught two fish.*

Use a comma **after an introductory phrase** or **adverbial clause**
Examples:
After the final out, we went to a restaurant to celebrate.
Studying the stars, I was surprised at the beauty of the sky.

Use a comma **between items in a series**
Example: I will bring *the turkey, the pie, and the coffee.*

The semicolon is used to connect major sentence pieces of equal value. Some rules for semicolons include:

Use a semicolon **between closely connected independent clauses** that are not connected with a coordinating conjunction.
Examples:
She is outside; we are inside.
You are right; we should go with your plan.

Use a semicolon **between independent clauses linked with a transitional word**.
Examples:
I think that we can agree on this; *however,* I am not sure about my friends.
You are looking in the wrong places; *therefore,* you will not find what you need.

Use a semicolon **between items in a series that has internal punctuation**.
Example: I have visited *New York, New York; Augusta, Maine; and Baltimore, Maryland.*

Use commas to **set off nouns of direct address, interrogative tags,** and **contrast**
Examples:
Direct Address: You, *John,* are my only hope in this moment.
Interrogative Tag: This is the last time, *correct*?
Contrast: You are my friend, *not my enemy.*

Use commas with **dates, addresses, geographical names,** and **titles**
Examples:
Date: *July 4, 1776,* is an important date to remember.
Address: He is meeting me at *456 Delaware Avenue, Washington, D.C.,* tomorrow morning.
Geographical Name: *Paris, France,* is my favorite city.
Title: John Smith, *Ph.D.,* will be visiting your class today.

Use commas to separate **expressions like *he said*** and ***she said*** if they come between a sentence of a quote
Examples:
"I want you to know," he began, "that I always wanted the best for you."
"You can start," Jane said, "with an apology."

English and Language Usage - Punctuation
© Mometrix Media - flashcardsecrets.com/teas
ATI TEAS Exam

Discuss the use of colons.

English and Language Usage - Punctuation
© Mometrix Media - flashcardsecrets.com/teas
ATI TEAS Exam

Discuss the use of parentheses.

English and Language Usage - Punctuation
© Mometrix Media - flashcardsecrets.com/teas
ATI TEAS Exam

Describe the use of quotation marks in quotations and in titles.

English and Language Usage - Punctuation
© Mometrix Media - flashcardsecrets.com/teas
ATI TEAS Exam

Discuss the use of quotation marks to indicate words being used ironically.

Visit *mometrix.com/academy* for a related video.
Enter video code: 884918

English and Language Usage - Punctuation
© Mometrix Media - flashcardsecrets.com/teas
ATI TEAS Exam

Discuss the placement of quotation marks in relation to periods, commas, semicolons, exclamation points, and question marks.

English and Language Usage - Punctuation
© Mometrix Media - flashcardsecrets.com/teas
ATI TEAS Exam

Describe the use of apostrophes.

Visit *mometrix.com/academy* for related videos.
Enter video codes: 213068 and 221438

Parentheses are used for additional information. Also, they can be used to put labels for letters or numbers in a series. Parentheses should not be used very often. If they are overused, parentheses can be a distraction instead of a help.

Examples:
Extra Information: The rattlesnake (see Image 2) is a dangerous snake of North and South America.
Series: Include in the email (1) your name, (2) your address, and (3) your question for the author.

The colon is used to call attention to the words that follow it. A colon must come after an **independent clause**. The rules for colons are as follows:

Use a colon **after an independent clause** to make a list
Example: I want to learn many languages: Spanish, French, German, and Italian.

Use a colon **for elaboration** or to **give a quote**
Examples:
Quote: The man started with an idea: "We are able to do more than we imagine."
Elaboration: There is one thing that stands out on your resume: responsibility.

Use a colon **after the greeting in a formal letter**, to **show hours and minutes**, and to **separate a title and subtitle**
Examples:
Greeting in a formal letter: Dear Sir: | To Whom It May Concern:
Time: It is 3:14 P.M.
Title: The essay is titled "America: A Short Introduction to a Modern Country"

Quotation marks may be used to set off words that are being used in a different way from a dictionary definition. Also, they can be used to highlight irony.

Examples:
The boss warned Frank that he was walking on "thin ice."
(Frank is not walking on real ice. Instead, Frank is being warned to avoid mistakes.)
The teacher thanked the young man for his "honesty."
(Honesty and truth are not always the same thing. In this example, the quotation marks around *honesty* show that the teacher does not believe the young man's explanation.)

Use quotation marks to close off **direct quotations** of a person's spoken or written words. Do not use quotation marks around indirect quotations. An indirect quotation gives someone's message without using the person's exact words. Use **single quotation marks** to close off a quotation inside a quotation.

Direct Quote: Nancy said, "I am waiting for Henry to arrive."
Indirect Quote: Henry said that he is going to be late to the meeting.
Quote inside a Quote: The teacher asked, "Has everyone read 'The Gift of the Magi'?"

Quotation marks should be used around the titles of **short works**: newspaper and magazine articles, poems, short stories, songs, television episodes, radio programs, and subdivisions of books or web sites.

Examples:
"Rip van Winkle" (short story by Washington Irving)
"O Captain! My Captain!" (poem by Walt Whitman)

An apostrophe is used to show **possession** or the deletion of letters in **contractions**. An apostrophe is not needed with the possessive pronouns *his, hers, its, ours, theirs, whose,* and *yours*.

Singular Nouns: David's car | a book's theme | my brother's board game
Plural Nouns with -s: the scissors' handle | boys' basketball
Plural Nouns without -s: Men's department | the people's adventure

Periods and commas are always put *inside* quotation marks. Colons and semicolons are always put *outside* quotation marks. Question marks and exclamation points are placed *inside* quotation marks when they are part of a quote. When the question or exclamation mark goes with the whole sentence, the mark is left *outside* of the quotation marks.

Examples:
Period and comma: We read "The Gift of the Magi," "The Skylight Room," and "The Cactus."
Semicolon: The class read "The Legend of Sleepy Hollow"; then they watched the movie adaptation.
Exclamation mark that is a part of a quote: The crowd cheered, "Victory!"
Question mark that goes with the whole sentence: Is your favorite short story "The Tell-Tale Heart"?

English and Language Usage - Punctuation

Describe the use of hyphens with compound words.

English and Language Usage - Punctuation

Describe the use of dashes in sentences.

English and Language Usage - Punctuation

Describe the use of an ellipsis.

English and Language Usage - Punctuation

Discuss the two main reasons to use brackets.

English and Language Usage - Improving Sentences

Discuss the rules for capitalization related to position in a sentence and proper nouns.

English and Language Usage - Improving Sentences

Discuss capitalization rules for directional names, titles of works, and kinship names.

Dashes are used to show a **break** or a **change in thought** in a sentence or to act as parentheses in a sentence. When typing, use two hyphens to make a dash. Do not put a space before or after the dash. The following are the rules for dashes:

To set off **parenthetical statements** or an **appositive with internal punctuation**
Example: The three trees—oak, pine, and magnolia—are coming on a truck tomorrow.

To show a **break or change in tone or thought**
Example: The first question—how silly of me—does not have a correct answer.

The hyphen is used in **compound words**. The following are the rules for hyphens:

Written-out numbers between 21 and 99 are written with a hyphen
Correct: *twenty-five* | one hundred *fifty-one* | *ninety-four* thousand
Incorrect: *seven-hundred* | *five-thousand* | *nine-teen*

Fractions need a hyphen if they are used as adjectives
Correct: The recipe says that we need a *three-fourths* cup of butter.
Incorrect: *One-fourth* of the road is under construction.

Compound words used as adjectives that come before a noun need a hyphen
Correct: The *well-fed* dog took a nap.
Incorrect: The dog was *well-fed* for his nap.

To **avoid confusion** with some words, use a hyphen
Examples: semi-irresponsible | Re-collect | Re-claim

Note: This is not a complete set of the rules for hyphens. A dictionary is the best tool for knowing if a compound word needs a hyphen.

There are two main reasons to use brackets:

When **placing parentheses inside of parentheses**
Example: The hero of this story, Paul Revere (a silversmith and industrialist [see Ch. 4]), rode through towns of Massachusetts to warn of advancing British troops.

When **adding explanation or details that are not part of a quote**
Example: The father explained, "My children are planning to attend my alma mater [State University]."

The ellipsis mark has three periods (…) to show when **words have been removed** from a quotation. If a full sentence or more is removed from a quoted passage, you need to use four periods to show the removed text and the end punctuation mark. The ellipsis mark should not be used at the beginning of a quotation. Also, the ellipsis should not be used at the end of a quotation. The exception is when some words have been deleted from the end of the final sentence.

Example:
"Then he picked up the groceries…paid for them…later he went home."

Capitalize directional names (north, east, south, west) **when they refer to specific areas**, but *not* **when they refer to the direction**
Examples:
Specific Area: James is from the *West*.
Direction: After three miles, turn *south* toward the highway.

Capitalize **all important words in a title** (articles, short prepositions, and short conjunctions are not capitalized unless they are the first or last word of the title)
Examples:
Correct: <u>Romeo and Juliet</u> is a beautiful drama on love.
Incorrect: <u>The Taming Of The Shrew</u> is my favorite. (Remember that internal prepositions and articles are not capitalized.)
Note: Books, movies, plays (more than one act), newspapers, magazines, and long musical pieces are put in italics. The two examples of Shakespeare's plays are underlined to show their use as an example.

Capitalize **kinship names** only if they are used as a **part or whole of a proper noun**. When using a kinship name descriptively, *do not* capitalize it.
Examples:
Kinship name as proper noun: Uncle Mark is coming over later tonight.
Kinship name as proper noun: Did you ask Mom if you could eat a cookie?
Descriptive kinship name: Sally 's uncle Jimbo is a ship captain.

The rules for capitalization are:
Capitalize the **first word of a sentence** and the **first word in a direct quotation**
Examples:
Sentence: *Football* is my favorite sport.
Direct Quote: She asked, "*What* is your name?"

Capitalize **proper nouns** and **adjectives that come from proper nouns**
Examples:
Proper Noun: My parents are from *Europe*.
Adjective from Proper Noun: My father is *British,* and my mother is *Italian*.

Capitalize the names of **days, months,** and **holidays**
Examples:
Day: Everyone needs to be here on *Wednesday*.
Month: I am so excited for *December*.
Holiday: *Independence Day* comes every July

English and Language Usage - Improving Sentences

Distinguish between the complete subject and the simple subject, and list a few situations in which the subject may be difficult to locate.

Visit *mometrix.com/academy* for a related video.
Enter video code: 444771

English and Language Usage - Improving Sentences

Identify the subject in each of the following sentences:
  John knows the way to the park.
  The cookies need ten more minutes.
  By five o' clock, Bill will need to leave.
  There are five letters on the table for him.
  There were coffee and doughnuts in the house.
  Go to the post office for me.
  Come and sit with me, please?

English and Language Usage - Improving Sentences

Define and discuss predicates and subjects.

English and Language Usage - Improving Sentences

Discuss subject verb agreement.

Visit *mometrix.com/academy* for a related video.
Enter video code: 479190

English and Language Usage - Improving Sentences

Give examples of subject-verb agreement for these special cases:
  words between the subject and the verb
  compound subject joined by *and*

English and Language Usage - Improving Sentences

Give examples of subject-verb agreement for these special cases:
  compound subject joined by *or*
  compound subject with *either/or*, *neither/nor*

Direct:
John knows the way to the park.
(Who knows the way to the park? Answer: John)
The cookies need ten more minutes.
(What needs ten minutes? Answer: The cookies)
By five o' clock, Bill will need to leave.
(Who needs to leave? Answer: Bill)

Remember: The subject can come after the verb.
There are five letters on the table for him.
(What is on the table? Answer: Five letters)
There were coffee and doughnuts in the house.
(What was in the house? Answer: Coffee and doughnuts)

Implied:
Go to the post office for me.
(Who is going to the post office? Answer: You are.)
Come and sit with me, please?
(Who needs to come and sit? Answer: You do.)

The subject of a sentence names who or what the sentence is about. The complete subject is composed of the **simple subject** and all of its **modifiers**.

To find the complete subject, ask *Who* or *What* and insert the verb to complete the question. The answer is the **complete subject**. To find the simple subject, remove all of the modifiers in the complete subject.
Examples:
The small red car is the one that he wants for Christmas.
(The complete subject is *the small red car*.)

The young artist is coming over for dinner.
(The complete subject is *the young artist*.)

In **imperative sentences**, the verb's subject is understood, but not actually present in the sentence. Although the subject ordinarily comes before the verb, in sentences that begin with *There are* or *There was*, the subject follows the verb. The ability to recognize the subject of a sentence helps in editing a variety of problems, such as sentence fragments and subject-verb agreement, as well as the using the correct pronouns.

Verbs agree with their subjects in **number**. In other words, singular subjects need singular verbs. Plural subjects need plural verbs. **Singular** is for one person, place, or thing. **Plural** is for more than one person, place, or thing. Subjects and verbs must also agree in person: first, second, or third. The present tense ending -s is used on a verb if its subject is third person singular; otherwise, the verb takes no ending.

Number Agreement Examples:
Single Subject and Verb: *Dan calls home.*
(Dan is one person. So, the singular verb *calls* is needed.)
Plural Subject and Verb: *Dan and Bob call home.*
(More than one person needs the plural verb *call*.)

Person Agreement Examples:
First Person: I *am* walking.
Second Person: You *are* walking.
Third Person: He *is* walking.

In a sentence, you always have a predicate and a subject. A **predicate** is what remains when you have found the subject. The **subject** tells what the sentence is about, and the predicate explains or describes the subject.

Think about the sentence: *He sings*. In this sentence, we have a subject (He) and a predicate (sings). This is all that is needed for a sentence to be complete. Would we like more information? Of course, we would like to know more. However, if this all the information that you are given, you have a complete sentence.

Now, let's look at another sentence:
John and Jane sing on Tuesday nights at the dance hall.
What is the subject of this sentence?
Answer: John and Jane.

What is the predicate of this sentence?
Answer: Everything else in the sentence besides John and Jane.

Today or tomorrow is the day.
(**Subject**: Today / tomorrow. **Verb**: is)

Stan or Phil wants to read the book.
(**Subject**: Stan / Phil. **Verb**: wants)

Neither the books nor the *pen is* on the desk.
(**Subject**: Books / Pen. **Verb**: is)

Either the blanket or *pillows arrive* this afternoon.
(**Subject**: Blanket / Pillows. **Verb**: arrive)

Note: Singular subjects that are joined with the conjunction *or* need a singular verb. However, when one subject is singular and another is plural, you make the verb agree with the **closer subject**. The example about books and the pen has a singular verb because the pen (singular subject) is closer to the verb.

Words between Subject and Verb
The joy of my life returns home tonight.
(**Singular Subject**: joy. **Singular Verb**: returns)
The phrase *of my life* does not influence the verb *returns*.

The question that still remains unanswered is "Who are you?"
(**Singular Subject**: question. **Singular Verb**: is)
Don't let the phrase "*that still remains…*" trouble you. The subject *question* goes with *is*.

Compound Subjects
You and Jon are invited to come to my house.
(**Plural Subject**: You and Jon. **Plural Verb**: are)

The pencil and paper belong to me.
(**Plural Subject**: pencil and paper. **Plural Verb**: belong)

Give examples of subject-verb agreement for these special cases:
    indefinite pronouns
    nouns formed from *every*, *any*

Discuss the use of collective nouns and relative pronouns as subjects.

Discuss nouns with plural form and singular meaning.

Discuss direct and indirect objects.

Discuss predicate nouns and predicate adjectives

Discuss pronoun-antecedents agreement.

Collective Nouns
The family eats at the restaurant every Friday night.
(The members of the family are one at the restaurant.)
The team are leaving for their homes after the game.
(The members of the team are leaving as individuals to go to their own homes.)

Who, Which, and That as Subject
This is the man *who* is helping me today.
He is a good man *who* serves others before himself.
This painting *that* is hung over the couch is very beautiful.

Indefinite Pronouns: Either, Neither, and Each
Is either of you ready for the game?
(**Singular Subject**: Either. **Singular Verb**: is)

Each man, woman, and child is unique.
(**Singular Subject**: Each. **Singular Verb**: is)

The adjective Every and compounds: Everybody, Everyone, Anybody, Anyone
Every day passes faster than the last.
(**Singular Subject**: Every day. **Singular Verb**: passes)

Anybody is welcome to bring a tent.
(**Singular Subject**: Anybody. **Singular Verb**: is)

Direct Objects
A direct object is a noun that takes or receives the **action** of a verb. Remember: a complete sentence does not need a direct object. A sentence needs only a subject and a verb. When you are looking for a direct object, find the verb and ask *who* or *what*.
Examples:
I took the blanket. (Who or what did I take? *The blanket*)
Jane read books. (Who or what does Jane read? *Books*)

Indirect Objects
An indirect object is a word or group of words that show how an action had an **influence** on someone or something. If there is an indirect object in a sentence, then you always have a direct object in the sentence. When you are looking for the indirect object, find the verb and ask *to/for whom or what*.
Examples:
We taught the old dog a new trick.
(To/For Whom or What was taught? *The old dog*)
I gave them a math lesson.
(To/For Whom or What was given? *Them*)

Plural Form and Singular Meaning
Some nouns are singular in meaning but plural in form: news, mathematics, physics, and economics
The news is coming on now.
Mathematics is my favorite class.

Some nouns are plural in meaning: athletics, gymnastics, scissors, and pants
Do these pants come with a shirt?
The scissors are for my project.

Note: Look to your dictionary for help when you aren't sure whether a noun with a plural form has a singular or plural meaning.
Addition, Multiplication, Subtraction, and Division are normally singular.
One plus one is two.
Three times three is nine

The **antecedent** is the noun that has been replaced by a pronoun. A pronoun and the antecedent agree when they have matching number and gender.

Singular agreement:
John came into town, and *he* played for us.
(The word *He* replaces *John*.)

Plural agreement:
John and Rick came into town, and *they* played for us.
(The word *They* replaces *John and Rick*.)

Predicate nouns are nouns that *modify the subject and finish linking verbs*.
Example: My father is a lawyer. (*Father* is the subject. *Lawyer* is the predicate noun.)

Predicate adjectives are adjectives that *modify the subject and finish linking verbs*.
Example: Your mother is patient. (*Mother* is the subject. *Patient* is the predicate adjective.)

English and Language Usage - Improving Sentences
© Mometrix Media - flashcardsecrets.com/teas
ATI TEAS Exam

Explain proper pronoun use in a compound subject or object.

Visit *mometrix.com/academy* for a related video.
Enter video code: 666500

English and Language Usage - Improving Sentences
© Mometrix Media - flashcardsecrets.com/teas
ATI TEAS Exam

Give an example to illustrate clear pronoun reference.

English and Language Usage - Improving Sentences
© Mometrix Media - flashcardsecrets.com/teas
ATI TEAS Exam

Explain how pronouns change form.

English and Language Usage - Improving Sentences
© Mometrix Media - flashcardsecrets.com/teas
ATI TEAS Exam

Explain the use of the words who and whom.

English and Language Usage - Improving Sentences
© Mometrix Media - flashcardsecrets.com/teas
ATI TEAS Exam

Discuss the two types of clauses.

English and Language Usage - Improving Sentences
© Mometrix Media - flashcardsecrets.com/teas
ATI TEAS Exam

Define and discuss the use of adjective clauses.

A pronoun should point clearly to the **antecedent**. Here is how a pronoun reference can be unhelpful if it is not directly stated or puzzling.

Unhelpful: Ron and Jim went to the store, and he bought soda.
(Who bought soda? Ron or Jim?)

Helpful: Jim went to the store, and he bought soda.
(The sentence is clear. Jim bought the soda.)

To determine the correct pronoun to use in a compound subject or object, try each pronoun separately in the sentence. Your knowledge of pronouns will tell you which one is correct.
Example: Bob and (I, me) will be going.
(Answer: Bob and I will be going.)

Test: (1) *I will be going* or (2) *Me will be going*. The second choice cannot be correct because *me* is not used as a subject of a sentence. Instead, *me* is used as an object.

When a pronoun is used with a noun immediately following (as in "we boys"), try the sentence without the added noun.
Example: (We/Us) boys played football last year.
(Answer: We boys played football last year.)

Test: (1) *We* played football last year or (2) *Us* played football last year. Again, the second choice cannot be correct because *us* is not used as a subject of a sentence. Instead, *us* is used as an object.

Who, a subjective-case pronoun, can be used as a subject. *Whom*, an objective case pronoun, can be used as an object. The words *who* and *whom* are common in **subordinate clauses** or in **questions**.

Subject: He knows *who* wants to come.
(*Who* is the subject of the verb *wants*.)

Object: He knows *whom* we want at the party.
(*Whom* is the object of *we want*.)

Some pronouns change their form by their placement in a sentence. A pronoun that is a subject in a sentence comes in the **subjective case**. Pronouns that serve as objects appear in the **objective case**. Finally, the pronouns that are used as possessives appear in the **possessive case**.

Subjective case: *He* is coming to the show.
(The pronoun *He* is the subject of the sentence.)

Objective case: Josh drove *him* to the airport.
(The pronoun *him* is the object of the sentence.)

Possessive case: The flowers are *mine*.
(The pronoun *mine* shows ownership of the flowers.)

An **adjective clause** is a dependent clause that modifies nouns and pronouns. Adjective clauses begin with a **relative pronoun** (*who, whose, whom, which,* and *that*) or a **relative adverb** (*where, when,* and *why*). Also, adjective clauses come after the noun that the clause needs to explain or rename. This is done to have a clear connection to the independent clause.

Examples:
I learned the reason why I won the award.
This is the place where I started my first job.

An adjective clause can be an essential or nonessential clause. An **essential clause** is very important to the sentence. Essential clauses explain or define a person or thing. **Nonessential clauses** give more information about a person or thing. However, they are not necessary to the sentence.

Examples:
Essential: A person *who works hard at first* can rest later in life.
Nonessential: Neil Armstrong, *who walked on the moon*, is my hero.

There are two types of clauses: independent and dependent. Unlike phrases, a **clause** has a subject and a verb. So, what is the difference between a clause that is independent and one that is dependent? An **independent clause** gives a complete thought. A **dependent clause** does not share a complete thought. Instead, a dependent clause has a subject and a verb, but it needs an independent clause. **Subordinate** (i.e., dependent) clauses look like sentences. They may have a subject, a verb, and objects or complements. They are used within sentences as adverbs, adjectives, or nouns.

Independent Clause: I am running outside. (Subject is *I* and verb is *am running*.)

Dependent Clause: I am running because I want to stay in shape.
The clause *I am running* is an independent clause. The underlined clause is dependent. Remember: a dependent clause does not give a complete thought. Think about the dependent clause: *because I want to stay in shape*.

Without any other information, you think: So, you want to stay in shape. What are you are doing to stay in shape? Answer: *I am running*.

Define and discuss the use of adverb clauses and noun clauses.

Define and discuss the use of phrases, including prepositional phrases.

Define and discuss the use of verbals including verbal phrases.

Describe the use of participles and participial phrases.

Define and discuss the use of gerunds and gerund phrases.

Discuss the use of infinitives and infinitive phrases.

A phrase is not a complete sentence; it cannot be a statement and cannot give a complete thought. Instead, a phrase is a group of words that can be used as a noun, adjective, or adverb in a sentence. Phrases strengthen sentences by *adding explanation or renaming something*.

Prepositional Phrases
A phrase that can be found in many sentences is the **prepositional phrase**. A prepositional phrase begins with a preposition and ends with a noun or pronoun that is used as an object. Normally, the prepositional phrase works as an adjective or an adverb.

Examples:
The picnic is *on the blanket*.
I am sick *with a fever* today.
Among the many flowers, a four-leaf clover was found by John.

An **adverb clause** is a dependent clause that modifies verbs, adjectives, and other adverbs. To show a clear connection to the independent clause, put the adverb clause immediately before or after the independent clause. An adverb clause can start with *after, although, as, as if, before, because, if, since, so, so that, unless, when, where*, or *while*.

Examples:
When you walked outside, I called the manager.
I want to go with you *unless you want to stay*.

A **noun clause** is a dependent clause that can be used as a subject, object, or complement. Noun clauses can begin with *how, that, what, whether, which, who,* or *why*. These words can also come with an adjective clause. Remember that the entire clause makes a noun or an adjective clause, not the word that starts a clause. So, be sure to look for more than the word that begins the clause. To show a clear connection to the independent clause, be sure that a noun clause comes after the verb. The exception is when the noun clause is the subject of the sentence.

Examples:
The fact that you were alone alarms me.
What you learn from each other depends on your honesty with others.

A participle is a verbal that is used as an adjective. The **present participle** always ends with *-ing*. **Past participles** end with *-d, -ed, -n,* or *-t*.

Examples: Verb: *dance* | Present Participle: *dancing* | Past Participle: *danced*

Participial phrases are made of a participle and any complements or modifiers. Often, they come right after the noun or pronoun that they modify.

Examples:
Shipwrecked on an island, the boys started to fish for food.
Having been seated for five hours, we got out of the car to stretch our legs.
Praised for their work, the group accepted the first-place trophy.

A verbal looks like a verb, but it is not used as a verb. Instead, a **verbal** is used as a noun, adjective, or adverb. Be careful with verbals. They do not replace a verb in a sentence.

Correct: Walk a mile daily.
(*Walk* is the verb of this sentence. As in, "*You* walk a mile daily.")
Incorrect: To walk a mile.
(*To walk* is a type of verbal. But, verbals cannot be a verb for a sentence.)

A **verbal phrase** is a verb form that does not function as the verb of a clause. There are three major types of verbal phrases: participial, gerund, and infinitive phrases.

An infinitive is a verbal that can be used as a noun, an adjective, or an adverb. An infinitive is made of the basic form of a verb with the word *to* coming before the verb.

Infinitive phrases are made of an infinitive and all complements and modifiers. They are used as nouns, adjectives, or adverbs.

Examples:
To join the team is my goal in life. (Noun)
The animals have enough food *to eat for the night*. (Adjective)
People lift weights *to exercise their muscles*. (Adverb)

A **gerund** is a verbal that is used as a noun. Gerunds can be found by looking for their *-ing* endings. However, you need to be careful that you have found a gerund, not a present participle. Since gerunds are nouns, they can be used as a subject of a sentence and the object of a verb or preposition.

Gerund phrases are built around present participles (i.e., *-ing* endings to verbs) and they are always used as nouns. The gerund phrase has a gerund and any complements or modifiers.

Examples:
We want to be known for *teaching the poor*. (Object of Preposition)
Coaching this team is the best job of my life. (Subject)
We like *practicing our songs* in the basement. (Object of the verb: *like*)

English and Language Usage - Improving Sentences

Define and discuss the use of appositives.

English and Language Usage - Improving Sentences

Define and discuss the use of absolute phrases.

English and Language Usage - Improving Sentences

List the five common modes of sentence patterns.

English and Language Usage - Improving Sentences

Discuss types of sentences.

English and Language Usage - Improving Sentences

Describe simple sentence structure.

English and Language Usage - Improving Sentences

Describe compound sentence structure and complex sentence structure.

Visit *mometrix.com/academy* for a related video.
Enter video code: 700478

An absolute phrase is a phrase with a participle that comes after a noun. The absolute phrase is never the subject of a sentence. Also, the phrase does not explain or add to the meaning of a word in a sentence. Absolute phrases are used *independently* from the rest of the sentence. However, they are still phrases, and a phrase cannot give a complete thought.

Examples:
The alarm ringing, he pushed the snooze button.
The music paused, she continued to dance through the crowd.

Note: Appositive and absolute phrases can be confusing in sentences. So, don't be discouraged if you have a difficult time with them.

An appositive is a word or phrase that is used to explain or rename nouns or pronouns. In a sentence they can be noun phrases, prepositional phrases, gerund phrases, or infinitive phrases.

Examples:
Terriers, *hunters at heart*, have been dressed up to look like lap dogs. (The phrase *hunters at heart* renames the noun *terriers*.)
His plan, *to save and invest his money*, was proven as a safe approach. (The italicized infinitive phrase renames the plan.)

Appositive phrases can be essential or nonessential. An appositive phrase is **essential** if the person, place, or thing being described or renamed is too general.

Essential: Two Founding Fathers George Washington and Thomas Jefferson served as presidents.
Nonessential: George Washington and Thomas Jefferson, two Founding Fathers, served as presidents.

For a sentence to be complete, it must have a subject and a verb or **predicate**. A complete sentence will express a complete thought, otherwise it is known as a **fragment**. An example of a fragment is: *As the clock struck midnight*. A complete sentence would be: *As the clock struck midnight, she ran home.* The types of sentences are declarative, imperative, interrogative, and exclamatory.

A **declarative sentence** states a fact and ends with a period.
Example: The football game starts at seven o'clock.

An **imperative sentence** tells someone to do something and ends with a period.
Example: Go to the store and buy milk.

An **interrogative sentence** asks a question and ends with a question mark.
Example: Are you going to the game on Friday?

An **exclamatory sentence** shows strong emotion and ends with an exclamation point.
Example: I can't believe we won the game!

Sentence patterns fall into five common modes with some exceptions. They are:
- Subject + linking verb + subject complement
- Subject + transitive verb + direct object
- Subject + transitive verb + indirect object + direct object
- Subject + transitive verb + direct object + object complement
- Subject + intransitive verb

Common exceptions to these patterns are questions and commands, sentences with delayed subjects, and passive transformations.

Compound Sentences – Compound sentences have two or more *independent clauses* with no dependent clauses. Usually, the independent clauses are joined with a comma and coordinating conjunction or with a semicolon.
Examples:
The time has come, and *we are ready*.
I woke up at dawn; then *I went outside to watch the sun rise*.

Complex Sentences – A complex sentence has one *independent clause* and one or more dependent clauses.
Examples:
Although he had the flu, Harry went to work.
Marcia got married after she finished college.

There are four major types of sentences: simple, compound, complex, and compound-complex.

Simple Sentences – Simple sentences have one Independent clause with no subordinate clauses. A simple sentence can have **compound elements** (e.g., a compound subject or verb).

Examples:
Judy *watered* the lawn. (single subject, single *verb*)
Judy and Alan *watered* the lawn. (compound subject, single *verb*)
Judy *watered* the lawn and *pulled* weeds. (single subject, compound *verb*)
Judy and Alan *watered* the lawn and *pulled* weeds. (compound subject, compound *verb*)

English and Language Usage - Improving Sentences
© Mometrix Media - flashcardsecrets.com/teas
ATI TEAS Exam

Describe compound-complex sentence structure.

English and Language Usage - Improving Sentences
© Mometrix Media - flashcardsecrets.com/teas
ATI TEAS Exam

Discuss sentence fragments.

Visit *mometrix.com/academy* for a related video.
Enter video code: 541989

English and Language Usage - Improving Sentences
© Mometrix Media - flashcardsecrets.com/teas
ATI TEAS Exam

Explain run on sentences and how to correct them.

English and Language Usage - Improving Sentences
© Mometrix Media - flashcardsecrets.com/teas
ATI TEAS Exam

Describe dangling modifiers and how to correct them.

English and Language Usage - Improving Sentences
© Mometrix Media - flashcardsecrets.com/teas
ATI TEAS Exam

Discuss modifiers and their uses.

English and Language Usage - Improving Sentences
© Mometrix Media - flashcardsecrets.com/teas
ATI TEAS Exam

Define and discuss split infinitives.

A part of a sentence should not be treated like a complete sentence. A sentence must be made of at least one **independent clause**. An independent clause has a subject and a verb. Remember that the independent clause can stand alone as a sentence. Some fragments are independent clauses that begin with a subordinating word (e.g., as, because, so, etc.). Other fragments may not have a subject, a verb, or both.

A **sentence fragment** can be repaired in several ways. One way is to put the fragment with a neighbor sentence. Another way is to be sure that punctuation is not needed. You can also turn the fragment into a sentence by adding any missing pieces. Sentence fragments are allowed for writers who want to show off their art. However, for your exam, sentence fragments are not allowed.

Fragment: Because he wanted to sail for Rome.
Sentence: He dreamed of Europe because he wanted to sail for Rome.

Compound-Complex Sentences – A compound-complex sentence has at least two *independent clauses* and at least one dependent clause.
Examples:
John is my friend who went to India, and *he brought souvenirs for us.*
You may not know, but *we heard the music* that you played last night.

A dangling modifier is a verbal phrase that does not have a clear connection to a word. A dangling modifier can also be a dependent clause (the subject and/or verb are not included) that does not have a clear connection to a word.

Examples:
Dangling: *Reading each magazine article*, the stories caught my attention.
Corrected: Reading each magazine article, *I* was entertained by the stories.
In this example, the word *stories* cannot be modified by *Reading each magazine article*. People can read, but stories cannot read. So, the pronoun *I* is needed for the modifying phrase *Reading each magazine article*.

Dangling: Since childhood, my grandparents have visited me for Christmas.
Corrected: Since childhood, I have been visited by my grandparents for Christmas.
In this example, the dependent adverb clause *Since childhood* cannot modify grandparents. So, the pronoun *I* is needed for the modifying adverb clause.

Run-on sentences consist of multiple independent clauses that have not been joined properly. Run-on sentences can be corrected in a variety of ways:

Joining the two independent clauses: Depending on how they are related, this could be done with a comma and coordinating conjunction, a semicolon, or a dash.
Incorrect: I went on the trip I had a good time.
Correct: I went on the trip, and I had a good time.

Changing one independent clause into a dependent clause: This is most easily done by simply adding a subordinating conjunction to the less important clause.
Incorrect: I went to the store I bought some eggs.
Correct: I went to the store where I bought some eggs.

Separating each independent clause into its own sentence: This correction is most effective when both independent clauses are long, or are not closely related. This can also be used when one sentence is a question and one is not.
Incorrect: I had pancakes for breakfast this morning they're my favorite.
Correct: I had pancakes for breakfast this morning. They're my favorite.

Reorganizing the thoughts in the sentence: This is often the best correction but requires the most work.
Incorrect: The drive to New York takes ten hours it makes me very tired.
Correct: During the ten-hour drive to New York, I get very tired.

A split infinitive occurs when a modifying word comes between the word *to* and the verb that pairs with *to*.

Example: To *clearly* explain vs. *To explain* clearly | To *softly* sing vs. *To sing* softly

Though still considered improper by some, split infinitives may provide better clarity and simplicity than the alternatives. As such, avoiding them should not be considered a universal rule.

In some sentences, a **modifier** can be put in more than one place. However, you need to be sure that there is no confusion about which word is being explained or given more detail.

Incorrect: He read the book to a crowd that was filled with beautiful pictures.
Correct: He read the book that was filled with beautiful pictures to a crowd.
The book was filled with beautiful pictures, not the crowd.

Incorrect: Derek saw a bus nearly hit a man on his way to work.
Correct: On his way to work, Derek saw a bus nearly hit a man.
Derek was on his way to work, not the other man.

English and Language Usage - Improving Sentences

Discuss the use of double negatives.

English and Language Usage - Improving Sentences

Explain the use of proper parallel structures in sentences.

English and Language Usage - Improving Sentences

Describe the use of subordinate clauses to show relative importance.

English and Language Usage - Improving Sentences

Explain the use of transitions in writing.

Visit *mometrix.com/academy* for a related video.
Enter video code: 707563

English and Language Usage - Improving Sentences

List some common transitional words that can be used to indicate the presence of examples or summaries.

English and Language Usage - Improving Sentences

List common transitional words that can be used to link similar ideas.

Parallel structures are used in sentences to highlight similar ideas and to connect sentences that give similar information. **Parallelism** pairs parts of speech, phrases, or clauses together with a matching piece. To write, *I enjoy reading and to study* would be incorrect. An infinitive does not match with a gerund. Instead, you should write *I enjoy reading and studying*.

Incorrect: He stopped at the office, grocery store, and the pharmacy before heading home.
Correct: He stopped at the office, *the* grocery store, and the pharmacy before heading home.

Incorrect: While vacationing in Europe, he went biking, skiing, and climbed mountains.
Correct: While vacationing in Europe, he went biking, skiing, and *mountain climbing*.

Standard English allows two negatives when a positive meaning is intended. For example, "The team was not displeased with their performance." **Double negatives** that are used to emphasize negation are not part of Standard English.

Negative modifiers (e.g., never, no, and not) should not be paired with other negative modifiers or negative words (e.g., none, nobody, nothing, or neither). The modifiers *hardly, barely*, and *scarcely* are also considered negatives in Standard English. So, they should not be used with other negatives.

Transitions are **bridges** between what has been read and what is about to be read. Transitions smooth the reader's path between sentences and inform the reader of major connections to new ideas forthcoming in the text. **Transitional phrases** should be used with care, selecting the appropriate phrase for a transition. **Tone** is another important consideration in using transitional phrases, and a good writer varies tone for different audiences. For example, in a scholarly essay, *in summary* would be preferable to the more informal *in short*.

When working with transitional words and phrases, writers usually find a natural **flow** that indicates when a transition is needed. In reading a draft of the text, it should become apparent where the flow is uneven or rough. At this point, the writer can add transitional elements during the revision process. **Revising** can also afford an opportunity to delete transitional devices that seem heavy handed or unnecessary.

When two items are not equal to each other, you can join them by making the more important piece an independent clause. The less important piece can become **subordinate**. To make the less important piece subordinate, you make it a phrase or a dependent clause. The piece of more importance should be the one that readers want or will need to remember.

Separated: The team had a perfect regular season. The team lost the championship.
Subordinated: Despite having a perfect regular season, *the team lost the championship*.

When a writer links ideas that are **similar** in nature, there are a variety of words and phrases he or she can choose, including but not limited to: *also, and, another, besides, equally important, further, furthermore, in addition, likewise, too, similarly, nor, of course,* and *for instance*.

Transitional words and phrases are used to transition between paragraphs and also to transition within a single paragraph. Transitions assist the flow of ideas and help to unify an essay. A writer can use certain words to indicate that an example or summary is being presented. The following phrases, among others, can be used as this type of transition: *as a result, as I have said, for example, for instance, in any case, in any event, in brief, in conclusion, in fact, in other words, in short, on the whole,* and *to sum it up*.

List common transitional words that can be used to link dissimilar or contradictory ideas.

List common transitional words that can be used to indicate cause, purpose, or result.

List common transitional words that can be used to indicate time or position.

Explain why tone is important in writing.

Discuss word usage.

Discuss the use of the words *which*, *that*, and *who*.

Visit *mometrix.com/academy* for a related video.
Enter video code: 197863

Writers may need to indicate that one thing is the **cause**, **purpose**, or **result** of another thing. To show this relationship, writers can use, among others, the following linking words and phrases: *as, as a result, because, consequently, hence, for, for this reason, since, so, then, thus,* and *therefore.*

Writers can link **contradictory** ideas in an essay by using, among others, the following words and phrases: *although, and yet, even if, conversely, but, however, otherwise, still, yet, instead, in spite of, nevertheless, on the contrary,* and *on the other hand.*

Tone may be defined as the writer's **attitude** toward the topic, and to the audience. This attitude is reflected in the language used in the writing. The tone of a work should be **appropriate** to the topic and to the intended audience. Some texts should not contain slang or **jargon**, although these may be fine in a different piece. Tone can range from humorous to serious and all levels in between. It may be more or less formal, depending on the purpose of the writing and its intended audience. All these nuances in tone can flavor the entire writing and should be kept in mind as the work evolves.

Certain words can be used to indicate the **time** and **position** of one thing in relation to another. Writers can use, for example, the following terms to create a timeline of events in an essay: *above, across, afterward, before, beyond, eventually, meanwhile, next, presently, around, at once, at the present time, finally, first, here, second, thereafter,* and *upon*. These words can show the order or placement of items or ideas in an essay.

The words *which*, *that*, and *who* can act as **relative pronouns** to help clarify or describe a noun.
Which is used for things only.
Example: Andrew's car, *which is old and rusty,* broke down last week.
That is used for people or things. *That* is usually informal when used to describe people.
Example: Is this the only book *that Louis L'Amour wrote?*
Example: Is Louis L'Amour the author *that wrote Western novels?*
Who is used for people or for animals that have a name.
Example: Mozart was the composer *who wrote those operas.*
Example: John's dog, *who is called Max,* is large and fierce.

Word usage, or **diction**, refers to the use of words with meanings and forms that are appropriate for the context and structure of a sentence. A common error in word usage occurs when a word's meaning does not fit the context of the sentence.

Incorrect: Susie likes chips better then candy.
Correct: Susie likes chips better than candy.

Incorrect: The cat licked it's coat.
Correct: The cat licked its coat.

Discuss the relationship between writer and reader.

Define and discuss clichés.

Define and discuss the use of jargon.

Discuss the use of slang.

Define and discuss the use of colloquialisms.

Define *point of view*, and list the three most common.

Clichés are phrases that have been **overused** to the point that the phrase has no importance or has lost the original meaning. The phrases have no originality and add very little to a passage. Therefore, most writers will avoid the use of clichés. Another option is to make changes to a cliché so that it is not predictable and empty of meaning.

Examples:
When life gives you lemons, make lemonade.
Every cloud has a silver lining.

The relationship between writer and reader is important in choosing a **level of formality** as most writing requires some degree of formality. **Formal writing** is for addressing a superior in a school or work environment. Business letters, textbooks, and newspapers use a moderate to high level of formality. **Informal writing** is appropriate for *private letters, personal e-mails, and business correspondence between close associates.*

For your exam, you will want to be aware of informal and formal writing. One way that this can be accomplished is to watch for shifts in point of view in the essay. For example, unless writers are using a personal example, they will rarely refer to themselves (e.g., "*I* think that *my* point is very clear.") to avoid being informal when they need to be formal.

Also, be mindful of an author who addresses his or her audience **directly** in their writing (e.g., "Readers, *like you*, will understand this argument.") as this can be a sign of informal writing. Good writers understand the need to be consistent with their level of formality. Shifts in levels of formality or point of view can confuse readers and discount the message of an author's writing.

Slang is an **informal** and sometimes private language that is understood by some individuals. Slang has some usefulness, but the language can have a small audience. So, most formal writing will not include this kind of language.

Examples:
"Yes, the event was a *blast*!" (the speaker means that the event was a great experience)
"That attempt was an *epic fail*." (the speaker means that the attempt was a spectacular failure.)

Jargon is a **specialized vocabulary** that is used among members of a trade or profession. Since jargon is understood by a small audience, writers tend to leave them to passages where certain readers will understand the vocabulary. Jargon includes exaggerated language that tries to impress rather than inform. Sentences filled with jargon are not precise and difficult to understand.

Examples:
"He is going to *toenail* these frames for us." (toenailing refers to nailing at an angle)
"They brought in a *kip* of material today." (a kip is a unit of measure equal to 1000 pounds)

Point of view is the **perspective** from which writing occurs. There are several possibilities:
- **First person** is written so that the *I* of the story is a participant or observer.
- **Second person** is written directly to the reader. is a device to draw the reader in more closely. It is really a variation or refinement of the first-person narrative.
- **Third person**, the most traditional form of point of view, is the omniscient narrator, in which the narrative voice, presumed to be the writer's, is presumed to know everything about the characters, plot, and action. Most writing uses this point of view.

A colloquialism is a word or phrase that is found in informal writing. Unlike slang, **colloquial language** will be familiar to a greater range of people. Colloquial language can include some slang, but these are limited to contractions for the most part.

Examples:
"Can *y'all* come back another time?" (y'all is a contraction of "you all")
"Will you stop him from building this *castle in the air*?" (A "castle in the air" is an improbable or unlikely event.)

Discuss the skills of writing and language usage in general.

Discuss the skill of brainstorming.

Describe free writing.

Discuss writing style.

Discuss revising sentences for the purposes of correcting errors and adding variety.

Discuss the recursive writing process.

Visit *mometrix.com/academy* for a related video.
Enter video code: 951611

Brainstorming is a technique that is used to find a creative approach to a subject. This can be accomplished by simple **free-association** with a topic. For example, with paper and pen, you write every thought that you have about the topic in a word or phrase. This is done without critical thinking. Everything that comes to your mind about the topic, you should put on your scratch paper. Then, you need to read the list over a few times. Next, you look for *patterns, repetitions, and clusters of ideas*. This allows a variety of fresh ideas to come as you think about the topic.

A writer's choice of words is a signature of their **style**. Careful thought about the use of words can improve a piece of writing. A passage can be an exciting piece to read when attention is given to the use of specific nouns rather than general ones.

Example:
General: His kindness will never be forgotten.

Specific: His thoughtful gifts and bear hugs will never be forgotten.

However you approach writing, you may find comfort in knowing that the revision process can occur in any order. The **recursive writing process** is not as difficult as the phrase may seem to indicate. Simply put, the recursive writing process means that you may need to revisit steps after completing other steps. Also implied in it is that there is no required order for the steps to take place. Indeed, you may find that **planning, drafting,** and **revising** (all a part of the writing process) take place at about the same time. The writing process involves moving back and forth between planning, drafting, and revising, and then more planning, more drafting, and more revising until the writing is satisfactory.

Writing is a skill that continues to need development throughout a person's life. For some people, writing seems to be a natural gift. They rarely struggle with writer's block. When you read their papers, you likely find their ideas persuasive. For others, writing is an intimidating task that they endure. As you prepare for the test, believe that you can improve your skills and be better prepared for reviewing several types of writing.

A traditional way to prepare for a test on language usage is to **read**. When you read newspapers, magazines, and books, you learn about new ideas. You can read newspapers and magazines to become informed about issues that affect many people. As you think about those issues and ideas, you can take a **position** and form **opinions**. Try to develop these ideas and your opinions by sharing them with friends. After you develop your opinions, try **writing** them down as if you were going to spread your ideas beyond your friends.

Remember that you are practicing for more than an exam. Two of the most valuable skills in life are the abilities to **read critically** and to **write clearly**. When you work on evaluating the arguments of a passage and explain your thoughts well, you are developing skills that you will use for a lifetime.

Free writing is a more structured form of brainstorming. The method involves a limited amount of time (e.g., 2 to 3 minutes) and writing everything that comes to mind about the topic in complete sentences. When time expires, you need to review everything that has been written down. Many of your sentences may make little or no sense, but the insights and observations that can come from free writing make this method a valuable approach. Usually, free writing results in a fuller expression of ideas than brainstorming because thoughts and associations are written in complete sentences. However, both techniques can be used to complement each other.

Revising sentences is done to make writing more effective. **Editing** sentences is done to correct any errors. Sentences are the building blocks of writing, and they can be changed in regards to sentence length, sentence structure, and sentence openings. You should add **variety** to sentence length, structure, and openings so that the essay does not seem boring or repetitive. A careful analysis of a piece of writing will expose these stylistic problems, and they can be corrected before you finish your essay. Changing up your sentence structure and sentence length can make your essay more inviting and appealing to readers.

English and Language Usage - Improving Paragraphs
© Mometrix Media - flashcardsecrets.com/teas
ATI TEAS Exam

Describe the structure of paragraphs in effective writing.

English and Language Usage - Improving Paragraphs
© Mometrix Media - flashcardsecrets.com/teas
ATI TEAS Exam

Discuss several ways that authors can support their arguments.

English and Language Usage - Improving Paragraphs
© Mometrix Media - flashcardsecrets.com/teas
ATI TEAS Exam

Discuss the different types of paragraphs that can be used.

English and Language Usage - Improving Paragraphs
© Mometrix Media - flashcardsecrets.com/teas
ATI TEAS Exam

Describe the use of different lengths of paragraphs.

English and Language Usage - Improving Paragraphs
© Mometrix Media - flashcardsecrets.com/teas
ATI TEAS Exam

Discuss some strategies used for making paragraphs coherent.

English and Language Usage - Vocabulary
© Mometrix Media - flashcardsecrets.com/teas
ATI TEAS Exam

Define context clues and explain how to use them.

A common method of development with paragraphs can be done with **examples**. These examples are the supporting details to the main idea of a paragraph or a passage. When authors write about something that their audience may not understand, they can provide an example to show their point. When authors write about something that is not easily accepted, they can give examples to prove their point.

Illustrations are extended examples that require several sentences. Well-selected illustrations can be a great way for authors to develop a point that may not be familiar to their audience.

Analogies make comparisons between items that appear to have nothing in common. Analogies are employed by writers to provoke fresh thoughts about a subject. These comparisons may be used to explain the unfamiliar, to clarify an abstract point, or to argue a point. Although analogies are effective *literary devices*, they should be used carefully in arguments. Two things may be alike in some respects but completely different in others.

Cause and effect is an excellent device used when the cause and effect are accepted as true. One way that authors can use cause and effect is to state the effect in the topic sentence of a paragraph and add the causes in the body of the paragraph. With this method, an author's paragraphs can have structure which always strengthens writing.

After the introduction of a passage, a series of **body paragraphs** will carry a message through to the conclusion. A paragraph should be unified around a **main point**. Normally, a good **topic sentence** summarizes the paragraph's main point. A topic sentence is a general sentence that introduces the paragraph.

The sentences that follow are a **support** to the topic sentence. However, the topic sentence can come as the final sentence to the paragraph if the earlier sentences give a clear explanation of the topic sentence. Overall, the paragraphs need to stay true to the main point. This means that any unnecessary sentences that do not advance the main point should be removed.

The **main point** of a paragraph requires adequate **development** (i.e., a substantial paragraph that covers the main point). A paragraph of only two or three sentences may not adequately cover a main point. An occasional short paragraph is fine as a **transitional device**. However, a well-developed argument will primarily consist of paragraphs with more than a few sentences.

Most readers find that their comfort level for a paragraph is *between 100 and 200 words*. Shorter paragraphs cause too much starting and stopping, and give a choppy effect. Paragraphs that are too long often test the attention span of readers. Two notable exceptions to this rule exist. In scientific or scholarly papers, longer paragraphs suggest seriousness and depth. In journalistic writing, constraints are placed on paragraph size by the narrow columns in a newspaper format.

The first and last paragraphs of a text will usually be the **introduction** and **conclusion**. These special-purpose paragraphs are likely to be shorter than paragraphs in the body of the work. Paragraphs in the body of the essay follow the subject's **outline**; one paragraph per point in short essays and a group of paragraphs per point in longer works. Some ideas require more development than others, so it is good for a writer to remain flexible. A paragraph of excessive length may be divided, and shorter ones may be combined.

A **paragraph of narration** tells a story or a part of a story. Normally, the sentences are arranged in chronological order (i.e., the order that the events happened). However, flashbacks (i.e., beginning the story at an earlier time) can be included.

A **descriptive paragraph** makes a verbal portrait of a person, place, or thing. When specific details are used that appeal to one or more of the senses (i.e., sight, sound, smell, taste, and touch), authors give readers a sense of being present in the moment.

A **process paragraph** is related to time order (i.e., First, you open the bottle. Second, you pour the liquid, etc.). Usually, this describes a process or teaches readers how to perform a process.

Comparing two things draws attention to their similarities and indicates a number of differences. When authors **contrast**, they focus only on differences. Both comparisons and contrasts may be used point-by-point or in following paragraphs.

Reasons for starting a new paragraph include:
- To mark off the introduction and concluding paragraphs
- To signal a shift to a new idea or topic
- To indicate an important shift in time or place
- To explain a point in additional detail
- To highlight a comparison, contrast, or cause and effect relationship

Learning new words is an important part of **comprehending** and **integrating** unfamiliar information. When a reader encounters a new word, he can stop and find it in the dictionary or the glossary of terms, but sometimes those reference tools aren't readily available or using them at the moment is impractical (e.g., during a test). Furthermore, most readers are usually not willing to take the time. Another way to determine the meaning of a word is by considering the **context** in which it is being used. These indirect learning hints are called **context clues**. They include definitions, descriptions, examples, and restatements. Because most words are learned by listening to conversations, people use this tool all the time even if they do it unconsciously. But to be effective in written text, context clues must be used judiciously because the unfamiliar word may have several subtle variations, and therefore the context clues could be misinterpreted.

A smooth flow of sentences and paragraphs without gaps, shifts, or bumps will lead to paragraph **coherence**. Ties between old and new information can be smoothed by several methods:

- **Linking ideas clearly**, from the topic sentence to the body of the paragraph, is essential for a smooth transition. The topic sentence states the main point, and this should be followed by specific details, examples, and illustrations that support the topic sentence. The support may be direct or indirect. In **indirect support**, the illustrations and examples may support a sentence that in turn supports the topic directly.
- The **repetition of key words** adds coherence to a paragraph. To avoid dull language, variations of the key words may be used.
- **Parallel structures** are often used within sentences to emphasize the similarity of ideas and connect sentences giving similar information.
- Maintaining a **consistent verb tense** throughout the paragraph helps. Shifting tenses affects the smooth flow of words and can disrupt the coherence of the paragraph.

Discuss context.

Visit *mometrix.com/academy* for a related video.
Enter video code: 613660

Define and discuss synonyms.

Define and discuss antonyms.

Visit *mometrix.com/academy* for a related video.
Enter video code: 105612

Discuss descriptive words in the text and how they can help you define unfamiliar words.

Discuss words that have more than one meaning.

Explain why understanding the structure of language is helpful to reading comprehension.

Visit *mometrix.com/academy* for a related video.
Enter video code: 894894

There are many pairs of words in English that can be considered **synonyms**, despite having slightly different definitions. For instance, the words *friendly* and *collegial* can both be used to describe a warm interpersonal relationship, and one would be correct to call them synonyms. However, *collegial* (kin to *colleague*) is often used in reference to professional or academic relationships, and *friendly* has no such connotation.

If the difference between the two words is too great, then they should not be called synonyms. *Hot* and *warm* are not synonyms because their meanings are too distinct. A good way to determine whether two words are synonyms is to substitute one word for the other word and verify that the meaning of the sentence has not changed. Substituting *warm* for *hot* in a sentence would convey a different meaning. Although warm and hot may seem close in meaning, warm generally means that the temperature is moderate, and hot generally means that the temperature is excessively high.

Context refers to *how a word is used in a sentence*. Identifying context can help determine the definition of unknown words. There are different contextual clues such as definition, description, example, comparison, and contrast. The following are examples:

- **Definition**: the unknown word is clearly defined by the previous words. – "When he was painting, his instrument was a ___." (paintbrush)
- **Description**: the unknown word is described by the previous words. – "I was hot, tired, and thirsty; I was ___." (dehydrated)
- **Example**: the unknown word is part of a series of examples. – "Water, soda, and ___ were the offered beverages." (coffee)
- **Comparison**: the unknown word is compared to another word. – "Barney is agreeable and happy like his ___ parents." (positive)
- **Contrast**: the unknown word is contrasted with another word. – "I prefer cold weather to ___ conditions." (hot)

Occasionally, you will be able to define an unfamiliar word by looking at the **descriptive words** in the context. Consider the following sentence: *Fred dragged the recalcitrant boy kicking and screaming up the stairs.* The words *dragged*, *kicking*, and *screaming* all suggest that the boy does not want to go up the stairs. The reader may assume that *recalcitrant* means something like unwilling or protesting. In this example, an unfamiliar adjective was identified.

Additionally, using description to define an unfamiliar noun is a common practice compared to unfamiliar adjectives, as in this sentence: *Don's wrinkled frown and constantly shaking fist identified him as a curmudgeon of the first order.* Don is described as having a *wrinkled frown and constantly shaking fist* suggesting that a *curmudgeon* must be a grumpy person. **Contrasts** do not always provide detailed information about the unfamiliar word, but they at least give the reader some clues.

Antonyms are words with opposite meanings. *Light* and *dark*, *up* and *down*, *right* and *left*, *good* and *bad*: these are all sets of antonyms. Be careful to distinguish between antonyms and pairs of words that are simply different. *Black* and *gray*, for instance, are not antonyms because gray is not the opposite of black. *Black* and *white*, on the other hand, are antonyms.

Not every word has an antonym. For instance, many nouns do not: What would be the antonym of chair? During your exam, any questions related to antonyms are more likely to concern adjectives. You will recall that adjectives are words that describe a noun. Some common adjectives include *purple*, *fast*, *skinny*, and *sweet*. From those four adjectives, *purple* is the item that lacks a group of obvious antonyms.

An understanding of the basics of language is helpful, and often vital, to understanding what you read. The term **structural analysis** refers to looking at the parts of a word and breaking it down into its different **components** to determine the word's meaning. Parts of a word include prefixes, suffixes, and the root word. By learning the meanings of prefixes, suffixes, and other word fundamentals, you can decipher the meaning of words which may not yet be in your vocabulary.

Prefixes are common letter combinations at the beginning of words, while **suffixes** are common letter combinations at the end. The main part of the word is known as the **root**. Visually, it would look like this: prefix + root word + suffix. Look first at the individual meanings of the root word, prefix and/or suffix. Using knowledge of the meaning(s) of the prefix and/or suffix to see what information it adds to the root.

Even if the meaning of the root is unknown, one can use knowledge of the prefix's and/or suffix's meaning(s) to determine an *approximate meaning* of the word. For example, if one sees the word *uninspired* and does not know what it means, they can use the knowledge that *un-* means 'not' to know that the full word means "not inspired." Understanding the common prefixes and suffixes can illuminate at least part of the meaning of an unfamiliar word.

When a word has **more than one meaning**, readers can have difficulty with determining how the word is being used in a given sentence. For instance, the verb *cleave*, can mean either *join* or *separate*. When readers come upon this word, they will have to select the definition that makes the most sense. Consider the following sentence: *Hermione's knife cleaved the bread cleanly.* Since, a knife cannot join bread together, the word must indicate separation.

A slightly more difficult example would be the sentence: *The birds cleaved together as they flew from the oak tree.* Immediately, the presence of the word *together* should suggest that in this sentence *cleave* is being used to mean *join*. Discovering the intent of a word with multiple meanings requires the same tricks as defining an unknown word: *look for contextual clues and evaluate the substituted words.*

English and Language Usage - Vocabulary

Discuss affixes and give the specific names for different types.

Visit *mometrix.com/academy* for a related video.
Enter video code: 782422

English and Language Usage - Vocabulary

Define and give examples of the following prefixes: bi-, mono-, poly-, semi-, and uni-.

English and Language Usage - Vocabulary

Define and give examples of the following prefixes: a-, in-, non-, and un-.

English and Language Usage - Vocabulary

Discuss some of the mechanical rules for adding suffixes to words.

English and Language Usage - Vocabulary

Explain suffixes and how they are used.

English and Language Usage - Vocabulary

Define and give examples of the following suffixes: -able (-ible), -esque, -ful, -ic, -ish, -less, and -ous.

Amount

Prefix	Definition	Examples
bi-	two	bisect, biennial
mono-	one, single	monogamy, monologue
poly-	many	polymorphous, polygamous
semi-	half, partly	semicircle, semicolon
uni-	one	uniform, unity

Affixes in the English language are **morphemes** that are added to words to create related but different words. **Derivational affixes** form new words based on and related to the original words. For example, the affix *–ness* added to the end of the adjective *happy* forms the noun *happiness*. **Inflectional affixes** form different grammatical versions of words. For example, the plural affix *–s* changes the singular noun *book* to the plural noun *books*, and the past tense affix *–ed* changes the infinitive or present tense verb *look* to the past tense *looked*.

Prefixes are affixes placed in front of words. For example, *heat* means to make hot; *preheat*, using the prefix *pre-*, means to heat in advance. **Suffixes** are affixes placed at the ends of words. The *happiness* example above contains the suffix *–ness*. **Circumfixes** add parts both before and after words, such as how *light* becomes *enlighten* with the prefix *en-* and the suffix *–en*. **Interfixes** compound words via central affixes: *speed* and *meter* become *speedometer* via the interfix *–o–*.

Suffixes are a group of letters, placed behind a root word, that carry a specific meaning. Suffixes can perform one of two possible functions. They can be used to create a new word, or they can shift the tense of a word without changing its original meaning. For example, the suffix *-ability* can be added to the end of the word *account* to form the new word *accountability*. *Account* means a written narrative or description of events, while *accountability* means the state of being liable. The suffix *-ed* can be added to *account* to form the word *accounted*, which simply shifts the word from present tense to past tense.

Negation

Prefix	Definition	Examples
a-	without, lacking	atheist, agnostic
in-	not, opposing	incapable, ineligible
non-	not	nonentity, nonsense
un-	not, reverse of	unhappy, unlock

Adjective Suffixes

Suffix	Definition	Examples
-able (-ible)	capable of being	toler*able*, ed*ible*
-esque	in the style of, like	picturesque, grotesque
-ful	filled with, marked by	thankful, zestful
-ic	make, cause	terrific, beatific
-ish	suggesting, like	churlish, childish
-less	lacking, without	hopeless, countless
-ous	marked by, given to	religious, riotous

Sometimes adding a suffix can change the **spelling** of a root word. If the suffix begins with a vowel, the final consonant of the root word must be doubled. This rule applies only if the root word has one syllable or if the accent is on the last syllable. For example, when adding the suffix *-ery* to the root word *rob*, the final word becomes *robbery*. The letter *b* is doubled because *rob* has only one syllable. However, when adding the suffix *-able* to the root word *profit*, the final word becomes *profitable*. The letter *t* is not doubled because the root word *profit* has two syllables.

Spelling is not changed when the suffixes *-less, -ness, -ly,* or *-en* are used. The only exception to this rule occurs when the suffix *-ness* or *-ly* is added to a root word ending in *y*. In this case, the *y* changes to *i*. For example, *happy* becomes *happily*.

English and Language Usage - Vocabulary
© Mometrix Media - flashcardsecrets.com/teas
ATI TEAS Exam

Define and give examples of the following suffixes: -ate, -en, fy, and -ize.

English and Language Usage - Vocabulary
© Mometrix Media - flashcardsecrets.com/teas
ATI TEAS Exam

Discuss suffixes with a modified root word.

English and Language Usage - Vocabulary
© Mometrix Media - flashcardsecrets.com/teas
ATI TEAS Exam

Define and give examples of the following prefixes: a-, ab-, ad-, ante-, anti-, cata-, circum-, com-, contra-, and de-.

English and Language Usage - Vocabulary
© Mometrix Media - flashcardsecrets.com/teas
ATI TEAS Exam

Define and give examples of the following prefixes: dia-, dis-, epi-, ex-, hypo-, inter-, intra-, ob-, per-, and peri-.

English and Language Usage - Vocabulary
© Mometrix Media - flashcardsecrets.com/teas
ATI TEAS Exam

Define and give examples of the following prefixes: post-, pre-, pro-, retro-, sub-, super-, and trans-.

English and Language Usage - Vocabulary
© Mometrix Media - flashcardsecrets.com/teas
ATI TEAS Exam

Define and give examples of the following prefixes: belli-, bene-, equi-, for-, fore-, homo-, hyper-, in-, magn-, mal-, mis-, and mor-.

Certain suffixes require that the root word be **modified**. If the suffix begins with a vowel, e.g., *-ing*, and the root word ends in the letter *e*, the *e* must be dropped before adding the suffix. For example, the word *write* becomes *writing*. If the suffix begins with a consonant instead of a vowel, the letter *e* at the end of the root word does not need to be dropped. For example, *hope* becomes *hopeless*. The only exceptions to this rule are the words *judgment, acknowledgment,* and *argument.* If a root word ends in the letter *y* and is preceded by a consonant, the *y* is changed to *i* before adding the suffix. This is true for all suffixes except those that begin with *i*. For example, *plenty* becomes *plentiful*.

Verb Suffixes

Suffix	Definition	Examples
-ate	having, showing	separate, desolate
-en	cause to be, become	deepen, strengthen
-fy	make, cause to have	glorify, fortify
-ize	cause to be, treat with	sterilize, mechanize, criticize

Time and Space Prefixes

Prefix	Definition	Examples
dia-	through, across, apart	diameter, diagnose
dis-	away, off, down, not	dissent, disappear
epi-	upon	epilogue
ex-	out	extract, excerpt
hypo-	under, beneath	hypodermic, hypothesis
inter-	among, between	intercede, interrupt
intra-	within	intramural, intrastate
ob-	against, opposing	objection
per-	through	perceive, permit
peri-	around	periscope, perimeter

Time and Space Prefixes

Prefix	Definition	Examples
a-	in, on, of, up, to	abed, afoot
ab-	from, away, off	abdicate, abjure
ad-	to, toward	advance, adventure
ante-	before, previous	antecedent, antedate
anti-	against, opposing	antipathy, antidote
cata-	down, away, thoroughly	catastrophe, cataclysm
circum-	around	circumspect, circumference
com-	with, together, very	commotion, complicate
contra-	against, opposing	contradict, contravene
de-	from	depart

Miscellaneous Prefixes

Prefix	Definition	Examples
belli-	war, warlike	bellicose
bene-	well, good	benefit, benefactor
equi-	equal	equivalent, equilibrium
for-	away, off, from	forget, forswear
fore-	previous	foretell, forefathers
homo-	same, equal	homogenized, homonym
hyper-	excessive, over	hypercritical, hypertension
in-	in, into	intrude, invade
magn-	large	magnitude, magnify
mal-	bad, poorly, not	malfunction, malpractice
mis-	bad, poorly, not	misspell, misfire
mor-	death	mortality, mortuary

Time and Space Prefixes

Prefix	Definition	Examples
post-	after, following	postpone, postscript
pre-	before, previous	prevent, preclude
pro-	forward, in place of	propel, pronoun
retro-	back, backward	retrospect, retrograde
sub-	under, beneath	subjugate, substitute
super-	above, extra	supersede, supernumerary
trans-	across, beyond, over	transact, transport

English and Language Usage - Vocabulary

Define and give examples of the following prefixes: neo-, omni-, ortho-, over-, pan-, para-, phil-, prim-, re-, sym-, and vis-.

English and Language Usage - Vocabulary

Define and give examples of the following suffixes: -acy, -ance, -ard, ation, -dom, -er(-or), -ess, -hood, and -ion.

English and Language Usage - Vocabulary

Define and give examples of the following prefixes: -ism, -ist, -ity(-ty), -ment, -ness, -ship, -sion(-tion), -th, and -tude.

Noun Suffixes

Suffix	Definition	Examples
-acy	state, condition	accuracy, privacy
-ance	act, condition, fact	acceptance, vigilance
-ard	one that does excessively	drunkard, sluggard
-ation	action, state, result	occupation, starvation
-dom	state, rank, condition	serfdom, wisdom
-er (-or)	office, action	teacher, elevator, honor
-ess	feminine	waitress, duchess
-hood	state, condition	manhood, statehood
-ion	action, result, state	union, fusion

Miscellaneous Prefixes

Prefix	Definition	Examples
neo-	new	Neolithic, neoconservative
omni-	all, everywhere	omniscient, omnivore
ortho-	right, straight	orthogonal, orthodox
over-	above	overbearing, oversight
pan-	all, entire	panorama, pandemonium
para-	beside, beyond	parallel, paradox
phil-	love, like	philosophy, philanthropic
prim-	first, early	primitive, primary
re-	backward, again	revoke, recur
sym-	with, together	sympathy, symphony
vis-	to see	visage, visible

Noun Suffixes

Suffix	Definition	Examples
-ism	act, manner, doctrine	barbarism, socialism
-ist	worker, follower	monopolist, socialist
-ity (-ty)	state, quality, condition	acidity, civility, royalty
-ment	result, action	refreshment, disappointment
-ness	quality, state	greatness, tallness
-ship	position	internship, statesmanship
-sion (-tion)	state, result	revision, expedition
-th	act, state, quality	warmth, width
-tude	quality, state, result	magnitude, fortitude